Central Sleep Apnea

Editors

CLODAGH M. RYAN
T. DOUGLAS BRADLEY

SLEEP MEDICINE CLINICS

www.sleep.theclinics.com

September 2026 • Volume 21 • Number 3

ELSEVIER

1818 Market Street • Suite 3323 • Philadelphia, Pennsylvania, 19103-2899

http://www.theclinics.com

SLEEP MEDICINE CLINICS Volume 21, Number 3
September 2026, ISSN 1556-407X, ISBN-13: 978-0-443-47044-8

Editor: Pat Manley
Developmental Editor: Akshay Samson

Publishing Office: *Sleep Medicine Clinics* (ISSN 1556-407X) is published quarterly by Elsevier Inc., 1818 Market Street, Philadelphia, PA 19103, United States. Periodicals postage paid at New York, NY and additional mailing offices. USA POSTMASTER: Send address changes to *Sleep Medicine Clinics*, Elsevier Customer Service Department, 3251 Riverport Lane, Maryland Heights, MO 63043, USA. Months of issue are March, June, September and December. Subscription prices are $271.00 per year (US individuals), $100.00 (US and Canadian students), $300.00 (Canadian individuals), $310.00 (international individuals), $135.00 (International students). For institutional access pricing please contact Customer Service via the contact information below. Foreign air speed delivery is included in all *Clinics* subscription prices. All prices are subject to change without notice. Orders, claims, and journal inquiries: Please visit our Support Hub page https://service.elsevier.com for assistance.

Reprints. For copies of 100 or more of articles in this publication, please contact the Commercial Reprints Department, Elsevier Inc., 360 Park Avenue South, New York, NY 10010-1710. Tel.: 212-633-3874; Fax: 212-633-3820; E-mail: reprints@elsevier.com.

Sleep Medicine Clinics is covered in *MEDLINE/PubMed (Index Medicus)*.

Printed by Sheridan at 450 Fame Avenue, Hanover, PA 17331.

SLEEP MEDICINE CLINICS

FORTHCOMING ISSUES

December 2026
Sleep Epileptology
Samson G. Khachatryan, *Editor*

March 2027
Artificial Intelligence in Sleep Medicine: From Algorithmic Promise to Clinical Reality
Ahmed S. BaHammam and Amir Sharafkhaneh, *Editors*

June 2027
Hypoventilation in Neuromuscular Disorders
Maju Pillai, *Editor*

RECENT ISSUES

June 2026
Sleep in Women
Naricha Chirakalwasan, *Editor*

March 2026
Sleep Disparities
Lourdes M. DelRosso, *Editor*

December 2025
Hospital Sleep Medicine and Non-Invasive Ventilation: emerging clinical paradigm
Michelle T. Cao, Robert C. Stansbury and Sunil Sharma, *Editors*

ISSUES OF RELATED INTEREST

Neurologic Clinics
https://www.neurologic.theclinics.com/

Contributors

CONSULTING EDITORS

TEOFILO LEE-CHIONG Jr, MD
Professor of Medicine, National Jewish Health, Professor of Medicine, University of Colorado, Denver, Colorado, USA; Chief Medical Liaison, Philips Respironics, Murrysville, Pennsylvania, USA

DIEGO GARCIA-BORREGUERO, MD, PhD
International Medical Director, Instituto del Sueño, Calle Padre Damián, Madrid, Spain

ANA C. KRIEGER, MD, MPH, FCCP, FAASM
Chief, Division of Sleep Neurology, Medical Director, Weill Cornell Center for Sleep Medicine, Professor of Clinical Medicine, Professor of Medicine in Neurology and Genetic Medicine, Weill Cornell Medical College, Cornell University, New York, New York, USA

EDITORS

CLODAGH M. RYAN, MB BChBAO, MD, FRCPC
Division of Respirology, Assistant Professor, Department of Medicine, University of Toronto, Sleep Research Laboratory, KITE Research Institute, Toronto Rehabilitation Institute, University Health Network, Toronto, Ontario, Canada

T. DOUGLAS BRADLEY, MD
Professor, Sleep Research Laboratory, Toronto Rehabilitation Institute, KITE Research Institute, Toronto General Hospital, Division of Respirology, Emeritus Professor, Department of Medicine, University Health Network, Sinai Health, University of Toronto, Toronto General Hospital Research Institute, Toronto, Ontario, Canada

AUTHORS

CHUN TING AU, RPSGT, PhD
Research Fellow, Translational Medicine, Research Institute, The Hospital for Sick Children, Toronto, Ontario, Canada

SÉBASTIEN BAILLIEUL, MD, PhD
Physiologist, Grenoble Alpes University, HP2 Laboratory, INSERM U1300, Grenoble Alpes University Hospital, Grenoble, France

MAYSAA BANJARI, MD
Neonatal Perinatal Fellow, Division of Neonatology, The Hospital for Sick Children, University of Toronto, Toronto, Ontario, Canada; Teaching Assistant, Department of Pediatrics, King Abdulaziz University, Jeddah, Saudi Arabia

T. DOUGLAS BRADLEY, MD
Professor, Sleep Research Laboratory, Toronto Rehabilitation Institute, KITE Research Institute, Toronto General Hospital, Division of Respirology, Emeritus Professor, Department of Medicine, University Health Network, Sinai Health, University of Toronto, Toronto General Hospital Research Institute, Toronto, Ontario, Canada

MARIA CASALINO, MD
Resident Physician, Department of Pediatrics, Queen's University, Kingston, Ontario, Canada

SAHAN CHANDRASEKARA, MBBS, FRACP
Fellow, Alfred Hospital, Melbourne, Victoria, Australia

MAIDA LYNN CHEN, MD
Professor of Pediatrics, Division of Pulmonary and Sleep, Seattle Children's Hospital, University of Washington School of Medicine, Seattle, Washington, USA

JULIANN M. DI FIORE, BS
Research Engineer III, Division of Neonatology, Department of Pediatrics, Rainbow Babies & Children's Hospital, Case Western Reserve University, Cleveland, Ohio, USA

ESTELLE B. GAUDA, MD
Professor, Department of Pediatrics, University of Toronto, Academic Lead, Division of Neonatology, University of Toronto, Senior Associate Scientist, Translational Medicine Program, SickKids Research Institute, Director, Toronto Centre for Neonatal Health, The Patient Support Center, The Hospital for Sick Children, Toronto, Ontario, Canada

RICHARD L. HORNER, PhD
Professor, Departments of Physiology and Medicine, University of Toronto, Toronto, Ontario, Canada

SAYAKI ISHIWATA, MD, PhD
Post-Doctoral Research Fellow, Sleep Research Laboratories of the University Health Network, Toronto Rehabilitation Institute (KITE), Toronto General Hospital, University of Toronto, Toronto, Ontario, Canada

OWEN D. LYONS, MB BChBAO, MCPI
Assistant Professor, Department of Medicine, Women's College Hospital, Women's College Research Institute, Sleep Research Laboratory, KITE-UHN, Toronto, Canada

KIMIHIKO MURASE, MD, PhD
Assistant Professor of Medicine, Department of Advanced Medicine for Respiratory Failure, Kyoto University Graduate School of Medicine, Kyoto University, Kyoto, Japan

INDRA NARANG, BMedSci, MBBCH, MD
Professor, Senior Associate Scientist, Department of Pediatrics, The Hospital for Sick Children, Toronto, Ontario, Canada

MATTHEW T. NAUGHTON, MD, FRACP
Head General Respiratory and Sleep Medicine, Alfred Hospital, Adjunct Professor of Medicine, Monash University, Victoria, Australia

ELISA PERGER, MD, PhD
Assistant Professor, Department of Medicine and Surgery, University of Milano-Bicocca, Istituto Auxologico Italiano, IRCCS, Sleep Disorders Center, Milan, Italy

CLODAGH M. RYAN, MB BChBAO, MD, FRCPC
Division of Respirology, Assistant Professor, Department of Medicine, University of Toronto, Sleep Research Laboratory, KITE Research Institute, Toronto Rehabilitation Institute, University Health Network, Toronto, Ontario, Canada

Contents

(ROHHAD) syndrome.In addition, the chapter examines related conditions such as Prader–Willi syndrome and other hypoventilation disorders arising from structural or functional abnormalities, including Chiari malformations and Leigh syndrome. It reviews current knowledge of the pathogenesis, epidemiology, clinical presentation, and diagnostic evaluation of these disorders in children, and concludes with evidence-based guidance for their management and treatment.

Preface
Central Sleep Apnea

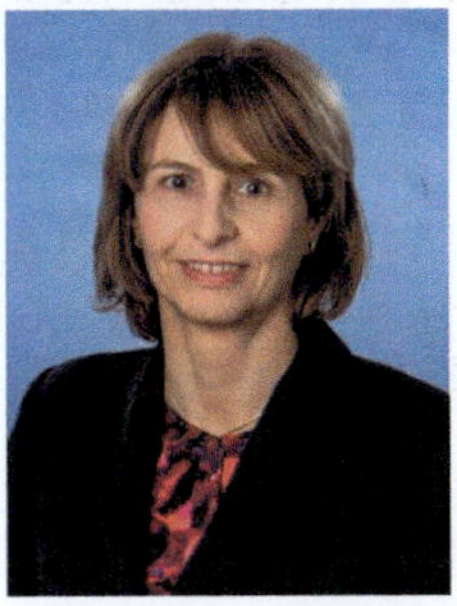

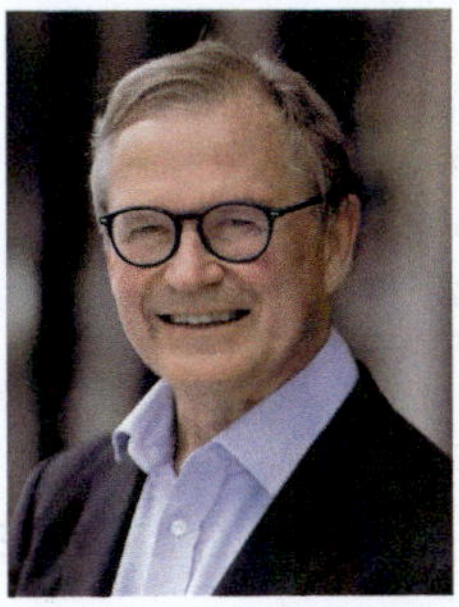

Clodagh M. Ryan, MB BChBAO, MD T. Douglas Bradley, MD
Editors

The original observations and description of central sleep apnea emanated from bedside medicine and go back to the late nineteenth century. John Cheyne's original 1818 publication "A Case of Apoplexy in Which the Flesh Part of the Heart Was Converted into Fat" was published in the *Dublin Hospital Reports*.[1] His bedside observations of a patient with heart failure is paraphrased from historical reviews: "the patient's respirations would cease entirely for a quarter of a minute or more, then become perceptible (though very low at first), gradually increase to a state of the highest effort, and then decline again until breathing ceased altogether, with this cycle repeating at regular intervals."[2] This definition provided the first description of the cyclical pattern of breathing with intermittent apneas and hyperpneas, which is recognizable today. In 1854, William Stokes independently reported this condition and expanded its description, specifically linking it to cardiac disease. These historical descriptions established that abnormal breathing could signal abnormalities in the regulation and control of circulatory and brain function, as well as blood-gas tensions that shaped subsequent clinical classification and research.[3]

The modern understanding of central sleep apnea emerged with the development of polysomnography in the late 1960s, but the formal classification did not occur until 1990 by the American Academy of Sleep Medicine. Over time, clinicians have recognized multiple related forms of central sleep apnea, linking it not only to heart failure but also to renal failure, strokes, opioid use, high altitude, and developmental disorders.

Bedside clinical medicine was the foundational rock upon which central sleep apnea was first described, and clinical presentation continues to guide our assessment and approach. While there continue to be gaps in our knowledge of

Sleep Med Clin 21 (2026) xi–xii
https://doi.org/10.1016/j.jsmc.2026.06.003
1556-407X/26/© 2026 Published by Elsevier Inc.

the pathophysiology of central sleep apnea, there has been significant progress over the last decade. This progress is attributable to combined efforts of clinician investigators, integrative physiologists, epidemiologists, and the participation of patient partners. Our objective in this issue was to provide clinicians with an updated overview of central sleep apnea and a clinical framework but also an in-depth understanding of current medical research on the pathophysiologic mechanisms underlying central sleep apnea, including current concepts on the control of breathing. The authors of these articles are experts in their respective fields and have made significant contributions to knowledge in this field.

Clodagh M. Ryan, MB BChBAO, MD
Sleep Research Laboratory
KITE Research Institute -
University Health Network
and Division of Respirology
Department of Medicine
University of Toronto
Toronto, Ontario, Canada

T. Douglas Bradley, MD
Sleep Research Laboratory
KITE Research Institute-
University Health Network
and Division of Respirology
Department of Medicine
University of Toronto
Toronto, Ontario, Canada

E-mail addresses:
clodagh.ryan@uhn.ca (C.M. Ryan)
douglas.bradley@utoronto.ca (T.D. Bradley)

REFERENCES

1. Cheyne J. A case of apoplexy in which the fleshy part of the heart was converted into fat. Dublin Hosp Rep 1818;2:216–23.
2. Lorenz R, Ito A. The definition of "Cheyne-Stokes rhythms. Acta Neurochir (Wien) 1978;43(1–2):61–76. https://doi.org/10.1007/BF01809226.
3. Guntheroth WG. Cheyne-Stokes respiration: hypoxia plus a deep breath that interrupts hypoxic drive, initiating cyclic breathing. Med Hypotheses 2011;77(5): 714–6. https://doi.org/10.1016/j.mehy.2011.07.023.

Control of Breathing

Richard L. Horner, PhD[a,b,*]

KEYWORDS

- Apnea • Arousal • Chemoreceptor • Hypercapnia • Hypoxia • Respiratory neurons
- Respiratory muscle • Sleep disorders

KEY POINTS

- This review first identifies the organization of the respiratory network to explain the differential effects of sleep on respiratory muscle activity and implications for breathing.
- The major factors and mechanisms influencing the efficacy of lung ventilation and control of blood gases are also identified, including the effects of sleep.
- The integrated respiratory and arousal responses to blood gas disturbances are discussed, including the predisposition to respiratory instability in sleep and therapeutic strategies.
- How these foundational physiologic principles that underpin the control of breathing apply to the spectrum of sleep-related breathing disorders is emphasized throughout.

INTRODUCTION

Apnea is identified by a temporary cessation of breathing. Apneas most commonly occur in sleep and are identified as (i) central apneas when there is no rhythmic drive to breath emanating from central respiratory neurons in the brainstem, hence leading to the absence of diaphragm activity and cessation of airflow; (ii) obstructive apneas when there is continuing breathing efforts but these are futile because of collapse of the pharyngeal airspace which prevents airflow into the lungs; and (iii) mixed apneas where a central apnea can precede an obstructive apnea and both can occur in the same event. All such apneas can lead to progressive hypoxia and hypercapnia during each event, and sleep disturbance. It is also the case that reduced central respiratory activity and/or partial pharyngeal closure can occur in sleep to produce periods of hypoventilation (ie, instead of outright apneas), together with clinically relevant blood gas disturbances and sleep disruption. It is an aim of this review to explain that such manifestations of apneas and hypopneas of the central and obstructive kinds share common principles and underlying mechanisms. Together, these common principles and underlying mechanisms of respiratory instability in sleep can be applied to the full spectrum of clinical sleep-related breathing problems.

ORGANIZATION OF CENTRAL RESPIRATORY ACTIVITY

Given that central apneas are defined by the temporary but repeated absence of the normal rhythmic drive to the muscles of breathing, the mechanisms underlying central respiratory activity are first identified.

Inspiration: Rhythmic respiratory drive arises from 2 main clusters of neurons in the medulla: the dorsal respiratory group (mainly inspiratory neurons) and the ventral respiratory group (inspiratory and expiratory neurons, with these mainly clustered in rostral and caudal regions respectively).[1–3] Contained within the rostral region of the ventral respiratory group is the pre-Bötzinger Complex that is thought essential to the generation of rhythmic respiratory activity in mammals.[4] First identified in a seminal study in rodents[4] in

[a] Department of Physiology, University of Toronto, 3206 Medical Sciences Building, 1 Kings College Circle, Toronto, Ontario M5S 1A8, Canada; [b] Department of Medicine, University of Toronto, 3206 Medical Sciences Building, 1 Kings College Circle, Toronto, Ontario M5S 1A8, Canada
* Corresponding author. Department of Physiology, University of Toronto, 3206 Medical Sciences Building, 1 Kings College Circle, Toronto, Ontario, M5S 1A8, Canada.
E-mail address: richard.horner@utoronto.ca

Sleep Med Clin 21 (2026) 287–298
https://doi.org/10.1016/j.jsmc.2026.05.001

Abbreviations	
CCHS	congenital central hypoventilation syndrome
CPAP	continuous positive airway pressure
FRC	functional residual capacity
NREM	nonrapid eye movement
PEEP	positive end-expiratory pressure
Phox2b	paired-like homeobox 2b

one of the most cited papers in respiratory physiology,[5] the pre-Bötzinger Complex is identified in humans.[6]

The key organizational principle of the central respiratory network is that the pre-Bötzinger Complex generates the fundamental respiratory rhythm and conveys this rhythmic activity to the inspiratory neurons of the dorsal and ventral respiratory groups. The dorsal and ventral respiratory groups then drive the activity of respiratory motoneurons in the spinal cord that innervate the respiratory pump muscles to generate airflow into the lungs. As such there is an important distinction between respiratory neurons of the pre-Bötzinger Complex and respiratory neurons of the dorsal and ventral respiratory groups: pre-Bötzinger Complex neurons are *proprio-bulbar* in that they project to other medullary respiratory neurons but *not* spinal respiratory motoneurons, whereas the dorsal and ventral respiratory groups are *bulbo-spinal* in that they activate spinal motoneurons to activate respiratory muscle.

Although pre-Bötzinger Complex neurons are proprio-bulbar and do not directly drive respiratory motoneurons and muscles, it would be incorrect to underestimate their importance as they are the key source of rhythmic drive to the whole respiratory network. Importantly, dysfunction of the pre-Bötzinger Complex caused by neurologic damage or drug-induced inactivation can lead to central apneas and uncoordinated breathing (ie, ataxic or Biot's breathing named after the French physician who, while an intern, differentiated this pattern from the distinctive waxing and waning pattern of Cheyne-Stokes breathing[7]).

Such dysfunction or cell loss in the pre-Bötzinger Complex can occur with aging or neurodegenerative diseases such as multiple system atrophy.[6] Dysfunction can also occur with neurodepressive drugs such as opioids because pre-Bötzinger Complex neurons express μ-opioid receptors[8,9] and the pre-Bötzinger Complex region is a major-site for opioid-induced respiratory depression.[10] Other respiratory neurons and motoneurons of the respiratory network also express μ-opioid receptors and contribute to respiratory depression.[11–14] It is notable that in the presence of dysfunction or cell loss of the pre-Bötzinger Complex that central apneas and ataxic breathing become especially apparent in sleep compared to wakefulness.[15,16] This phenomenon introduces the concept that the presence of wakefulness itself can provide sufficient excitatory drive to the respiratory system to mask (at least partially) otherwise important defects in respiratory control. The clinical relevance is that sedating agents and opioid drugs can seem well tolerated in the initially alert patient but, when the stimulating effects of wakefulness are withdrawn, the patient can suffer major respiratory depression. Pharmacologic strategies to target the stimulation of pre-Bötzinger Complex neurons, or to preserve their activity and prevent opioid-induced respiratory depression, ataxic breathing and central apneas while selectively preserving analgesia, is an area of active research with clinical implications.[17,18]

Expiration: There are 3 main clusters of expiratory neurons in the medulla: (i) Bötzinger Complex neurons that are rostral to the inspiratory neurons of the pre-Bötzinger Complex; (ii) parafacial expiratory neurons located nearby the facial motor nucleus and in the vicinity of the Bötzinger Complex; and (iii) the caudal region of the ventral respiratory group. This latter group contains the bulbo-spinal neurons that directly drive the expiratory intercostal and abdominal muscles of breathing. Importantly, excitation of these central expiratory neurons during resting breathing does not necessarily manifest as measurable expiratory muscle activation. Nevertheless, during situations of increased respiratory drive, including during sleep, expiratory neurons and expiratory muscles are actively recruited and this can contribute to increased ventilation, and stabilization of breathing and reduced apneas.[19–21]

The expiratory muscles are typically tonically active during resting stable breathing, and this importantly contributes to the maintenance of functional residual capacity (FRC). Given that phasic, respiratory-related, expiratory muscle activity is typically not observed during resting breathing, the lung deflation that occurs in expiration is normally *passive*. This is because the lungs, due to their inherent elasticity, naturally recoil after their expansion during inspiration. It is for this reason that positive end-expiratory pressure (PEEP) and continuous positive airway pressure (CPAP) act to increase FRC by virtue of the positive airway pressure at end-expiration opposing this passive elastic-recoil. As reviewed in a later section, this effect of PEEP and CPAP can have important stabilizing effects on breathing in several sleep-related breathing disorders beyond obstructive sleep apnea.

CENTRAL RESPIRATORY ACTIVITY AND PRINCIPLES ARISING

Two foundational concepts in respiratory physiology are: (i) central respiratory neurons vary in the strength of their relationship to breathing, and (ii) there is a differential effect of sleep on their activities. These features can explain the signature changes in respiratory muscle activities across sleep-wake states that ultimately give rise to sleep-related breathing disorders.

Central respiratory neurons vary in the strength and consistency of their relationship to breathing: The strength and consistency of the activity of a respiratory neuron to breathing and airflow can be formally quantified by the *eta-squared statistic* (η^2), with values ranging from 0 to 1 (weak to strong). The interpretation of the η^2 values of respiratory neurons is best understood from the original paper[22]: (i) high η^2 cells are *quintessentially respiratory..., protected from non-respiratory distortions, ... because of rigid sequences of excitatory and inhibitory postsynaptic potentials that preclude activity that is not strictly respiratory*—that is, those neurons that are strongly influenced by the respiratory oscillator and weakly by other nonrespiratory, tonic, inputs; (ii) in contrast, the activity of *low η2-valued cells is the apparent result of mixtures of inputs that have respiratory and nonrespiratory forms*, that is, those more strongly influenced by nonrespiratory tonic inputs than breathing per se.[22]

Signature effects of sleep: Cardinal features of central respiratory neurons and the effects of sleep upon them are (i) central respiratory neurons are differentially sleep sensitive, (ii) with *high* η2 neurons being *least* affected by the transition to nonrapid eye movement (NREM) sleep such that there is relative preservation of their activity, and (iii) *low* η2 neurons being *most* affected by NREM sleep such that their activity significantly decreases or even ceases, (iv) with some inspiratory neurons being *activated* in rapid eye movement (REM) sleep even in the presence of hypocapnia that was otherwise sufficient to silence their respiratory activity in NREM sleep, that is, spontaneous breathing can reappear in REM sleep despite hypocapnia.[22,23]

Principles arising: As identified in the preceding section, sleep has differential effects in suppressing the activity of low versus high η^2 respiratory neurons.[24–26] There are several manifestations of these fundamental effects that are relevant to both normal physiology and pathophysiology.

Firstly, different respiratory muscles have different levels of respiratory and tonic activities, and this is because of the innervations they receive from the central respiratory neurons that drive them. As such, some muscles are mainly tonically active during resting breathing such as the tensor palatini of the soft palate, whereas others express both tonic and respiratory activities such as the tongue and the intercostal muscles, while the diaphragm is exclusively respiratory during breathing.

Secondly, that low η2 neurons are most affected by NREM sleep explains the particularly sleep-sensitive nature of tonic respiratory muscle activity, and the consequent signature reductions in tonic palatal, tongue and intercostal muscle activities that occur at sleep onset. The decreased tonic activity of those central respiratory neurons that ultimately drive the pharyngeal muscles are responsible for the normal increase in upper airway resistance in sleep, with this being a major contributor to the hypoventilation and elevated $Pa{CO_2}$ observed in sleep compared to wakefulness.[27–29]

Thirdly, the decreased tonic activity of central respiratory neurons leads to reduced tonic activity of the chest wall muscles, which in turn leads to normal decreases in FRC of 200 to 500 mL in sleep compared to waking.[30] In supine individuals with obesity, the mass loading of the chest exacerbates the decreased FRC. These effects are not without consequence. Firstly, the decreased lung volume increases upper airway resistance due to reduced caudal traction (*tug*) of the trachea; reduced *tug* increases pharyngeal wall thickness and narrows the airspace predisposing to collapse and obstructive apneas.[31] Secondly, reduced tonic activity of the intercostal muscles also contributes to hypoventilation in sleep, especially REM sleep, as the motor neurons are less excitable during inspiration.[2] This hypoventilation becomes especially apparent in patients who rely on chest wall activity for adequate lung ventilation such as those with those with diaphragm dysfunction or weakness.[32,33] Over time there is evidence of plasticity and inspiratory recruitment of nondiaphragmatic accessory respiratory muscles in REM sleep to help sustain breathing in some patients with diaphragm paralysis.[34]

There is a fourth, and significant, consequence of this normal decreased FRC in sleep that predisposes to unstable breathing and apneas.[31] Smaller lung volumes contribute to a reduced total volume of gases stored in the body such that any given change in lung ventilation produces larger swings in $Pa{O_2}$ and $Pa{CO_2}$. This in turn elicits larger oscillations in ventilation that manifests as unstable breathing in sleep with cyclical periods of hyperventilation, hypoventilation, and apneas. In control system terminology as related to breathing, such a reduced lung volume increases *plant gain*: a situation where a given change in ventilation is more effective in eliminating CO_2 and can precipitate apnea.[31] This effect will be a focus at the conclusion of this article to bring all these concepts together.

Wakefulness stimulus to breathing and predisposition to hypoventilation in sleep: A continuous, background excitatory drive that tonically stimulates the central respiratory network and motor outflow to the respiratory muscles in wakefulness, but whose influence is withdrawn at sleep onset, is a long-standing concept in respiratory physiology and sleep medicine.[35–37] This wakefulness-dependent tonic excitation into the respiratory network is termed the *wakefulness stimulus* and/or *behavioral influence*. Both terms have been used interchangeably and encompass wakefulness-dependent mechanisms that affect breathing whether one is aware of them or not, and whether they are volitional or not.

Activity of the low $\eta 2$ respiratory neurons is essentially the neural substrate for the 'wakefulness stimulus' to breathing and the tonic activity of those low $\eta 2$ neurons is due to the collective activity of the brain arousal systems of wakefulness.[35–37] The withdrawal at sleep onset of this wakefulness-dependent tonic excitation into the respiratory network leaves the network critically dependent on the remaining source of tonic drive into the system to provide *enough* excitation to sustain rhythmic breathing and prevent apnea. This second source of tonic drive is from the central and peripheral chemoreceptors. As such, adequate breathing becomes critically dependent in sleep on the feedback regulation in sleep provided by the chemoreceptors.[2] The influence of tonic chemoreceptor drive derives largely from the central chemoreceptors, with a nontrivial $\sim$10% of this tonic chemoreceptor drive arising from the peripheral chemoreceptors at the carotid bodies.[38,39]

Critical dependence of breathing on chemoreceptor feedback in sleep: The clinical relevance of this reliance on tonic chemoreceptor drive in sleep to sustain effective breathing is that *any* defect in chemoreceptor function can precipitate significant hypoventilation in sleep when the wakefulness stimulus to breathing is withdrawn. This functional organization explains why, for example, individuals with chronic low awake Pa_{CO_2} (eg, in congestive heart failure) or deficient CO_2-sensing brain chemosensors (eg, in congenital central hypoventilation syndrome, CCHS) can experience significant central apneas and/or hypopneas in NREM sleep resulting in recurrent hypoxemia, sleep disturbance, and potentially the failure to wake up from sleep in the case of CCHS.[40–45] Notably, however, the heightened state of brain arousal in REM sleep (or wakefulness) can provide a level of tonic excitatory input of sufficient magnitude to restore or replace the *wakefulness stimulus/behavioral influence* and reinstate breathing. It is because of this effect of REM sleep that central apneas and hypoventilation are less prevalent, or not present, in REM sleep compared to NREM sleep in such patients with congestive heart failure or CCHS.[40–46]

In this context of CCHS, a major breakthrough in respiratory physiology was the identification and subsequent phenotyping of those CO_2/H^+-sensitive neurons in the medulla that comprise the central chemoreceptors. The central chemoreceptors are located in the retrotrapezoid nucleus, with their cell bodies situated below the ventral surface of the medulla but with their dendrites and sensory endings extending to the surface in close association with circulating cerebrospinal fluid to detect changes in pH due to changes in CO_2.[47–49] The link to CCHS deserves additional comment. Mutations in the paired-like homeobox 2b (Phox2b) gene, a gene expressed in central and peripheral chemoreceptor neurons, has been identified in over 99% of CCHS patients.[2,46] Although CCHS is typically identified in newborns, it can also present in adults and is due to another Phox2b mutation.[44] Such individuals can survive to adulthood without early respiratory failure and not require ventilatory support during sleep until diagnosis. However, subtle signs and symptoms can be exhibited during childhood such as unusually long breath-hold times with no respiratory discomfort, and unexplained seizures.[44] Overall, that Phox2b is expressed in chemoreceptor neurons and not in respiratory neurons is thought to explain the ability of CCHS patients to breathe adequately when awake, that is, the brainstem systems generating respiratory rhythm and output are not defunct, rather that wakefulness per se can provide sufficient excitatory drive to mask the major defect in chemoreceptor function caused by the Phox2b mutation. The ability of CCHS patients to also breathe in REM sleep further reinforces the principle that the state of central nervous system excitation that is an inherent feature of REM sleep can also provide sufficient excitation to the central respiratory network for the generation of breathing.

CHEMORECEPTOR MECHANISMS AND RESPONSES IN SLEEP

Central chemoreceptors—location and action: CO_2-sensitive retrotrapezoid neurons are taken to be *the* central chemoreceptors because they fulfill a set of criteria including being intrinsically responsive to H^+/CO_2, able to detect small changes in pH, and stimulate breathing via axon projections to the ventral respiratory group.[47–49] Other brainstem neurons can also be activated by CO_2, indirectly in some cases, but do not necessarily fulfill all the criteria to be intrinsically responsive to CO_2 and thereby function as specialized central chemoreceptors.[47,50] Such neurons include serotonergic raphe neurons, and noradrenergic neurons of the locus coeruleus that are integral to sleep–wake circuitry in that they contribute to the brain arousal of wakefulness and have reduced activity in sleep.[2,50–57] All such neurons are positioned to contribute to the full manifestation of the ventilatory response to hypercapnia by their projections to the respiratory network and its motor outputs including the upper airway, chest wall and diaphragm, including the important arousal response to chemoreceptor stimulation.[2,58]

The blood brain barrier is relatively impermeable to polar solutes such as H^+ and HCO_3^- so systemic changes in H^+, as can occur with metabolic acidosis, do not directly influence the pH of the cerebrospinal fluid.[2] In such a situation of metabolic acidosis, the stimulation of breathing is via the peripheral chemoreceptors. In contrast, CO_2 itself diffuses rapidly and freely across the blood brain barrier and subsequently decreases the pH in the cerebrospinal fluid to stimulate sensory afferents of retrotrapezoid chemoreceptor neurons. Given the location of the retrotrapezoid neurons, these central chemoreceptors are relatively slow to respond to a change in Pa_{CO_2}, with up to ~30 sec to begin the breathing response and up to 5 min to respond fully and achieve steady-state.[38]

Ventilatory response to hypercapnia and effects of sleep: The ventilatory response to hypercapnia is quantified as the change in ventilation resulting from a dynamic increase in Pa_{CO_2} produced by rebreathing at a constant Pa_{O_2}, or via stepwise, steady-state, changes in Pa_{CO_2}. In humans, the average slope (ie, sensitivity) of the hypercapnic ventilatory response markedly decreases from wakefulness to NREM sleep to REM sleep (~1.6 to ~0.8 to ~0.5 $L.min^{-1}.mm\ Hg^{-1}$ respectively).[59] It is noted that although these are average values, there is a wide range (up to 6-fold) of the ventilatory response to hypercapnia between individuals.

Peripheral chemoreceptors—location, action, and modulation: The peripheral chemoreceptors are located in the carotid and aortic bodies, with the carotid bodies being the strongly dominant of the two in mammals, especially humans.[60,61] The carotid bodies, located at the bifurcation of the common carotid arteries, receive one of the highest blood supplies per tissue weight in the body.[60] Given the location of the carotid bodies between the brain and the heart and lungs, these chemoreceptors are positioned to respond rapidly to a change in blood gases: within 10 sec in individuals with normal circulation compared to, for example, ~25 sec in patients with congestive heart failure and Cheyne-Stokes breathing with central apneas.[39,40] In routine clinical scenarios this time lag can be estimated as the *lung to ear circulation time*, which is an indirect measure of the circulatory delay from the onset of a first breath after an apnea (ie, reoxygenation of the lungs) to the measured increase in arterial oxygen levels from its nadir as measured by an ear oximeter that is at approximately the same level as the carotid bodies.[40]

The carotid bodies respond to both changes in Pa_{O_2} and Pa_{CO_2} to effectively function as *asphyxia* receptors. Carotid body activity increases with increased Pa_{CO_2}, with an increased slope of response (ie, increased sensitivity) and leftward shift of response (ie, decreased threshold) as the levels of Pa_{O_2} decline.[62,63] As such, hypoxia significantly sensitizes the peripheral chemoreceptor response to hypercapnia. The peripheral chemoreceptors are effectively silenced in 100% O_2,[62] and the resulting immediate decrease in ventilation can be used to assess the relative contribution of the peripheral chemoreceptors to resting breathing, a test known as the *Dejours Test* after the French physician Pierre Dejours.[39]

The mechanisms of O_2 sensing by the carotid body, and the sensitization by CO_2, is complex and somewhat outside the scope of this review but are simplified and briefly summarized here to give insight into how and why some respiratory stimulants are used clinically, including for central and obstructive sleep apnea. In short, there are multiple O_2 sensors in the carotid body including a variety of heme containing proteins and O_2 sensitive K^+ channels that provide for sensory responsiveness over a wide range of O_2 affinities (eg, Pa_{O_2} of 80–20 mm Hg) and rapidity of responses (<1 sec) respectively.[64] Chemosensory glomus cells in the carotid body express many types of neurotransmitters and synapse with afferent nerve endings whose cell bodies are in the petrosal ganglion, with afferent inputs to the brain via the carotid branch of the glossopharyngeal nerve (carotid sinus nerve).[65] Ultimately, hypoxia and hypercapnia inhibit pH-sensitive background K^+ leak channels to cause depolarization of the chemosensory glomus cells.[66,67] This leads to increased intracellular Ca^{2+} via voltage gated Ca^{2+}entry, and exocytosis of neurotransmitter including adenosine triphosphate and acetylcholine. These excite and depolarize the afferent nerve endings and the transmission of chemosensory information to the nucleus of the tractus solitarius and the initiation of the effector responses.

It is with this mechanism and context that the use of K^+ channel blockers has some utility in modulating peripheral chemoreceptor responses for respiratory disorders. Doxapram is an inhibitor of pH-sensitive background K^+ leak channels,[68] and its respiratory stimulant properties are thought to arise from effects at the carotid body chemoreceptors to increase their activity by mimicking the effects of hypoxia and hypercapnia on the same channels.[66,67] The effects of carbonic anhydrase inhibitors such as acetazolamide and sulthiame are somewhat complicated but are thought to induce bicarbonaturea via renal effects, and thereby a metabolic acidosis to stimulate breathing, again via effects at the peripheral chemoreceptors given that the blood brain barrier is relatively impermeable to polar solutes.[69]

Ventilatory response to hypoxia and effects of sleep: The ventilatory response to hypoxia is quantified as the change in ventilation following changes in oxygen saturation (SaO_2) or Pao_2. In humans, the average slope (sensitivity) of the response markedly decreases from wakefulness to NREM and REM sleep ($\sim$1.0 to $\sim$0.6 to $\sim$0.3 $L.min^{-1}.\%SaO_2^{-1}$ respectively).[70]

Impaired blood gases in wakefulness are always worse in sleep: A generalizable principle in respiratory medicine is that any disorder that impairs breathing and blood gases in wakefulness typically leads to significant worsening of blood gases in sleep.[2,32,37,71] In healthy individuals, the normal reductions in lung ventilation from wakefulness to sleep normally leads to trivial reductions in arterial oxygen saturation because of the starting position on the upper flat part of the oxy-hemoglobin dissociation curve. In individuals with compromised lung function and blood gases in wakefulness, it is expected that there would be significant decreases in arterial oxygen saturation in sleep as they are closer to, or already on, the steep portion of the oxy-hemoglobin dissociation curve given the sigmoidal relationship of Po_2 and oxygen saturation.[2]

Arousal responses to blood gas disturbances in sleep: In the case of hypoventilation in sleep, the appropriate physiologic response includes both a chemoreceptor-mediated increase in ventilation and arousal from sleep. The latter can be particularly relevant in the face of significantly deteriorating hypoventilation.[37,58,72,73] Asphyxia resulting from an obstruction to breathing (eg, obstructive sleep apnea), breathing depression (eg, with opioids), impaired lung function, or suffocation (eg, sleeping face down) can all eventually elicit arousal from sleep. Such arousal responses are dampened in REM sleep compared to NREM.[2,37]

The brain mechanisms of arousal from sleep in response to blood gas disturbances have received significant attention in recent years. Some cell groups are positioned to modulate the integrated respiratory and arousal responses to hypercapnia including pontine serotonergic, noradrenergic and glutamate neurons that are intimately involved in sleep–wake regulation.[53–57,74–81] Of note are the glutamatergic neurons in the parabrachial nucleus given their recent identification as the key neuronal hub mediating the respiratory and arousal responses to hypercapnia.[74–78] Given their important role in the integrated arousal and ventilatory responses, these sleep-wake modulating cell groups are also a source of vulnerability because any decrements in their function, for example, caused by sedation[82–87] and/or hypoxic cell damage,[88] can impair the ventilatory and alerting responses. Failure to respond to worsening asphyxia is thought responsible for some unexpected deaths in Sudden Infant Death Syndrome, sleep apnea, and after accidental mismanagement of sedatives and opioids.[2] Between 25% and 50% of the deaths attributed to Sudden Infant Death Syndrome are thought to be due to face-down rebreathing asphyxia resulting from sleeping conditions such as soft surface bedding and cosleeping.[72,89]

INTEGRATIVE RESPIRATORY CONTROL ACROSS SLEEP–WAKE STATES AND PREDISPOSITION TO INSTABILITY AND APNEAS

In the terminology of the control system for breathing, the sensitivity of the ventilatory response to blood gas disturbances is termed *controller gain*. In this context, the *controller* includes all the chemosensory, neural and anatomic contributors (eg, upper airway and respiratory pump muscles) that together comprise the ventilatory responses to hypercapnia and hypoxia.[31] This is only one side of the relationship between ventilation and blood gas homeostasis, the other being *plant gain*. The 'plant' is the total volume of gases stored in the body, and as such it includes the FRC.[31] Overall, plant gain reflects the effectiveness of a change in ventilation to alter blood gases, whereas a change in blood gases will itself lead to a change in ventilation with the sensitivity of that response being controller gain. The sum of the plant and controller gains comprises total *loop gain*.

A high gain system responds quickly and vigorously to a perturbation, whereas a low gain system responds slowly and weakly. For the control of breathing, common perturbations or disturbances to breathing include a transient hyperventilation or hypoventilation caused by a sigh, a respiratory pause or apnea, or a transition from wakefulness to sleep or vice versa. In any of these common situations, the breathing disturbance alters blood gases, which then leads to a ventilatory response, which itself then alters blood gases, which then leads to a ventilatory response and so on. If loop gain is less than 1 then the response and subsequent disturbances and responses get progressively smaller and diminish over time, such that breathing stabilizes and returns to equilibrium. If loop gain is ≥ 1 then the response to the disturbance is equal or greater than the disturbance itself such that the instability and oscillations in breathing persist and manifest as cyclical hyperventilation and hypoventilation, and repetitive apneas.[31,90] This unstable breathing pattern will continue until some new factor breaks the cycle: for example, changing body position to lessen the chances of an obstructive apnea, a return to wakefulness, deeper NREM sleep, or a transition to REM sleep.

It is this predisposition to instability that explains the common observation in patients with sleep apnea that they do not necessarily have apneas all of the time in sleep.[31,90] For example, patients with Cheyne-Stokes respiration due to heart failure commonly exhibit high loop gain and low awake $Paco_2$, but they can have periods of stable breathing in NREM sleep.[2,31,40,90] However, arousal from sleep can trigger a transient hyperventilation followed by subsequent hypocapnia that can precipitate repetitive central sleep apneas in NREM thereafter, with prolonged circulatory delay also playing an important role in determining apnea cycle length.[40] Nevertheless, the central apneas can disappear in REM sleep as the nonspecific excitatory 'behavioral influences' on the respiratory system return in REM sleep, and because $Paco_2$ can increase as the ventilatory responses to altered blood gases are blunted in REM sleep (ie, the controller gain component of loop gain decreases), and the disturbing effect of arousal from sleep is also reduced compared to NREM sleep.[2,40] Likewise, obstructive apneas can be absent for prolonged periods, with deeper NREM sleep being both a consequence of less apneas as well as contributing to less apneas because the threshold to elicit arousal from sleep is also raised and stable sleep predisposes to stable breathing.[90]

Fig. 1 illustrates how the concepts discussed in this review all interact to predispose to unstable breathing and how therapeutic strategies can stabilize the system. The equilibrium point for resting breathing can be taken for the purposes of this discussion as $\sim$5.5 $L.min^{-1}$ with a $Paco_2$ of $\sim$40 mm Hg. **Fig. 1** shows that during steady-state metabolism, the equilibrium for resting breathing is situated at the intersection of the response of ventilation to a change in $Paco_2$, and the response of $Paco_2$ to a change in ventilation.[31] Any transient disturbances in breathing and normal variations lead to constant resettling around the equilibrium (see **Fig. 1**).

The response of $Paco_2$ to a change in ventilation is defined by the relationship of alveolar (and hence arterial) Pco_2 for a given ventilation at the prevailing metabolic rate: $Paco_2$ (mm Hg) $\propto$ metabolic CO_2 production (eg, 250 $mL.min^{-1}$)/alveolar ventilation (eg, 5.4 $L.min^{-1}$).[31] The constant of proportionality with these units is 0.863. This relationship is termed the "*metabolic hyperbola*", with the tangent at any point indicating the effectiveness of ventilation to eliminate CO_2 (ie, δ $Paco_2$ in response to a given δ ventilation which reflects plant gain, see **Fig. 1**A). Given the shape of this relationship, a shift toward hyperventilation or increased lung volume reflects a lower plant gain as a larger change in ventilation is needed to produce a given change in $Paco_2$, whereas a shift toward hypoventilation or decreased lung volume reflects a higher plant gain as a smaller change in ventilation is needed to produce the same change in $Paco_2$ (see **Fig. 1**).[2,31,90]

Reductions in $Paco_2$ below eupnea reduce ventilation according to the ventilatory response (controller gain) until apnea develops, and the $Paco_2$ at which this occurs is termed the "*apnea threshold*" (see **Fig. 1**).[2,31,90] The apnea threshold is readily observed in NREM sleep because ventilation is dependent on chemoreceptor activity in the absence of the 'wakefulness stimulus'/ 'behavioral influences' on breathing, but these influences can be present and sufficiently stimulate breathing despite hypocapnia in wakefulness and REM sleep.

The magnitude of an increase in ventilation that is sufficient to lower $Paco_2$ to the apnea threshold is termed the *CO_2 reserve* (see **Fig. 1**).[2,31,90] The inherent predisposition to unstable breathing is therefore based upon the relative proximity of the equilibrium $Paco_2$ to the apnea threshold, or how easily the CO_2 reserve is depleted to reach this threshold.[2,31,90] Decreases in plant and/or controller gains produce a scenario whereby a larger ventilatory disturbance is necessary to deplete the CO_2 reserve and elicit hypopnea and apnea (see **Fig. 1**).[2,31,90] The opposite occurs with increases in plant and/or controller gains, that is, a smaller ventilatory disturbance is sufficient to deplete the CO_2 reserve and elicit hypopnea and apnea.[2,31,90]

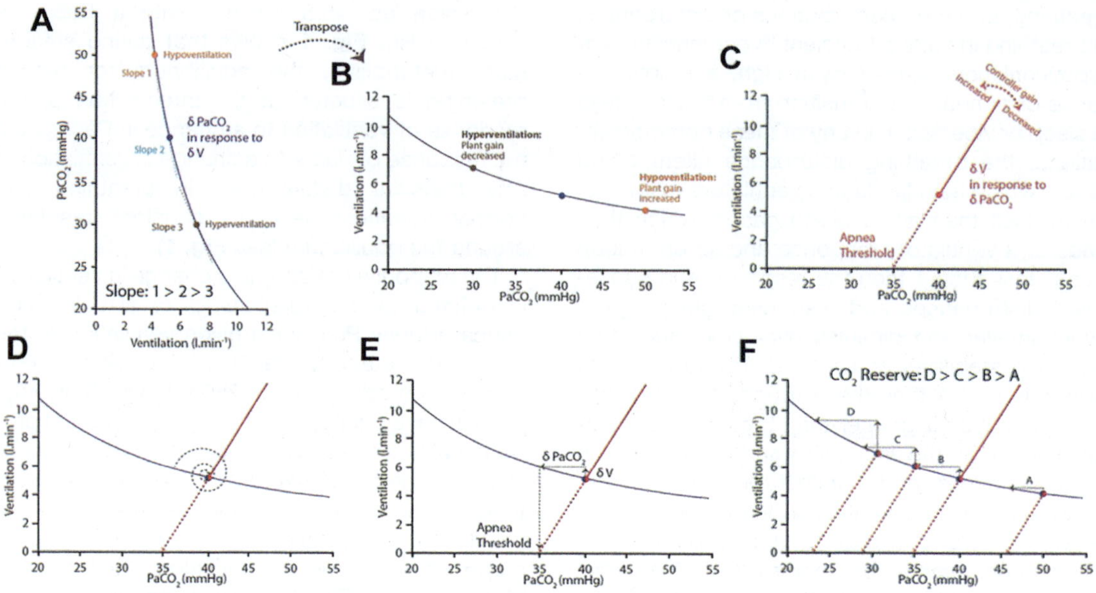

Fig. 1. (*A*) The metabolic hyperbola (*blue line*) identifies the change in Pa_{CO_2} that results from a change in alveolar ventilation. Eupnea is shown with a Pa_{CO_2} of ~40 mm Hg and an alveolar ventilation of ~5.4 $L.min^{-1}$ (*blue circular symbol*) The 3 tangents shown intersecting with the metabolic hyperbola at conditions of hypoventilation (*orange symbol*), eupnea (*blue symbol*), and hyperventilation (*brown symbol*) represent the effectiveness of ventilation to eliminate CO_2 (ie, plant gain). Note that the plant gain progressively decreases from hypoventilation to eupnea to hyperventilation (represented by slopes 1, 2 and 3). The relationship (*A*) is then transposed (*B*) to allow for subsequent superimposition with the ventilatory response to increased arterial P_{CO_2} (*C*). The change in ventilation that results from a change in Pa_{CO_2} (ie, controller gain) is shown above eupnea (*red circular symbol* and *solid red line*) and below eupnea (*dashed line*). The level of hypocapnia at which ventilation ceases is the apnea threshold. Note that decreasing the controller gain around the same eupneic Pa_{CO_2} and ventilation would lower the apnea threshold, whereas increasing the controller gain would increase the apnea threshold closer to the eupneic Pa_{CO_2}. The equilibrium point for resting breathing sits at the intersection of the metabolic hyperbola and the ventilatory response to CO_2 (see *mixed red and blue symbols D–F*), with any transient disturbances in breathing leading to constant resettling around the equilibrium (see *spiral* in *D*). Any transient increase in ventilation (δV, indicated by the *upward dashed black line* and *arrow*) will reduce Pa_{CO_2} (δ$PaCO_2$ indicated by the *leftward black arrow*) according to the metabolic hyperbola, and elicit an apnea if the resultant hypocapnia reaches the apnea threshold as extrapolated from the ventilatory response to CO_2 (*E*). The CO_2 reserve is the magnitude of the δ$PaCO_2$ required to reach the apnea threshold. Note that progressive leftward shifts on the metabolic hyperbola leads to progressive increases in the CO_2 reserve, whereas a rightward shift decreases the CO_2 reserve (*F*). Ultimately breathing in sleep is more stable and resilient to transient perturbations in ventilation with a larger CO_2 reserve. See text for further details.

The culmination of these interactions is foundational physiologic principles in respiratory control: (i) the predisposition to stable or unstable breathing in sleep is significantly determined by plant and controller gains, and (ii) these gains can be specifically targeted for therapeutic effect. Interventions such as PEEP and CPAP increase FRC and dead space, thereby effectively reducing plant gain.[2,31,90] With the larger total volume of gases stored in the body, any given change in lung ventilation produces smaller oscillations in arterial P_{CO_2} and the resulting smaller resulting oscillations in ventilation show as more stable breathing in sleep. Interventions such as hyperoxia can reduce peripheral chemoreceptor responsiveness and thus controller gain.[62,63] Reductions in plant gain and/or controller gain effectively increase the CO_2 reserve and so make it less likely to be depleted and thus the apnea threshold less likely to be reached (see **Fig. 1**). It is also for this reason that patients with chronic alveolar hypoventilation secondary to central nervous system dysfunction or neuromuscular weakness are predisposed to periodic breathing in sleep despite having an elevated Pa_{CO_2} as the position on the metabolic hyperbola reflects a higher plant gain, that is, a relatively small change in ventilation can deplete the CO_2 reserve and so elicit hypoventilation and apnea.[2] Likewise, patients with congestive heart failure that have sympathetic nervous system-mediated increases in controller gain that lower awake Pa_{CO_2} are also predisposed to hypocapnic central sleep apneas as the apnea threshold is already reached at the transition to NREM sleep.[2,40]

This article concludes with one more example as it relates to the treatment of periodic breathing in sleep as it nicely highlights the interaction of plant and controller gains given that it is difficult to influence one and not the other. Carbonic anhydrase inhibitors such as acetazolamide and sulthiame are thought to produce a metabolic acidosis and peripheral chemoreceptor-induced respiratory stimulation that may be involved in them significantly reducing breathing instability and sleep apnea severity.[69,91,92] Meta-analyses and model simulations suggest that the positive effects on breathing instability and sleep apnea severity are most strongly linked to decreases in plant gain that dominate potential increases in controller gain caused by the metabolic acidosis: for example, plant gain can decrease by ~32% with carbonic anhydrase inhibitions due to a leftward shift on the metabolic hyperbola (see **Fig. 1**) such that overall loop gain decreases by ~26%.[69] In this scenario, the higher level of ventilation on the metabolic hyperbola leads to a lower plant gain with a larger CO_2 reserve, and thus breathing is more stable with the overall reduced loop gain[69] (see **Fig. 1**).

Although high loop gain is the key mechanism typically linked to the pathogenesis of central sleep apnea it is also a significant contributor to obstructive apneas.[31,93–95] Such a strong effect of effect of carbonic anhydrase inhibitors such as acetazolamide and sulthiame on lowering overall loop gain can explain the improvements in obstructive sleep apnea severity in recent studies.[69,91,92,96] Improving pharyngeal muscle activity and responsiveness, upper airway collapsibility, and the destabilizing effects of arousal from sleep are also targets to reduce sleep apnea severity clinically but their detailing is outside the scope of this review focusing on the control of breathing more generally, and other topical sources are suggested for the interested reader.[93,97–103]

CLINICS CARE POINTS

- Identification of the major physiologic principles that are the foundation of the control of breathing during sleep can explain the spectrum of clinical sleep-related breathing disorders, especially the predisposition to respiratory instability that characterizes central and obstructive apneas.
- This understanding is also the basis for current treatment strategies that target specific pathophysiological mechanisms.
- Such mechanisms encompass core concepts such as loop gain that is comprised of controller and plant gains. These are identified and explained, and effective strategies to target them are identified including proof-of principle clinical interventions and studies.

FUNDING

This article was funded by the Canadian Institutes of Health Research, Canada (CIHR, Grant PJT-180288 and PJT-153243), and the National Sanitarium Association Innovative Research Program (fund number 00144051).

DISCLOSURE

The author has nothing to disclose.

REFERENCES

1. Del Negro CA, Funk GD, Feldman JL. Breathing matters. Nat Rev Neurosci 2018;19(6):351–67.
2. Horner RL, Malhotra A. Control of breathing and upper airways during sleep. In: Broaddus VC, Ernst JD, King TE Jr, et al, editors. Murray & Nadel's textbook of respiratory medicine. 7th edition. Philadelphia (PA): Elsevier; 2022. p. 1618–32. chap 117.
3. Horner RL. Respiratory physiology. In: Kushida CA, editor. Encyclopedia of sleep and circadian rhythms. 2nd edition. Amsterdam, Netherlands: Elsevier, Academic Press; 2023. p. 200–9.
4. Smith JC, Ellenberger HH, Ballanyi K, et al. Pre-Botzinger complex: a brainstem region that may generate respiratory rhythm in mammals. Science 1991;254(5032):726–9.
5. Fitzgerald RS, Cherniack NS. Historical perspectives on the control of breathing. Compr Physiol 2012;2(2):915–32.
6. Schwarzacher SW, Rub U, Deller T. Neuroanatomical characteristics of the human pre-botzinger complex and its involvement in neurodegenerative brainstem diseases. Brain 2011;134(Pt 1):24–35.
7. Wijdicks EF. Biot's breathing. J Neurol Neurosurg Psychiatry 2007;78(5):512–3.
8. Gray PA, Janczewski WA, Mellen N, et al. Normal breathing requires preBotzinger complex neurokinin-1 receptor-expressing neurons. Nat Neurosci 2001; 4(9):927–30.
9. Gray PA, Rekling JC, Bocchiaro CM, et al. Modulation of respiratory frequency by peptidergic input to rhythmogenic neurons in the preBotzinger complex. Science 1999;286(5444):1566–8.
10. Montandon G, Qin W, Liu H, et al. PreBötzinger complex neurokinin-1 receptor-expressing neurons

mediate opioid-induced respiratory depression. J Neurosci 2011;31:1292–301.
11. McCrimmon DR, Alheid GF. On the opiate trail of respiratory depression. Am J Physiol 2003;285(6): R1274–5.
12. McCrimmon DR, Zuperku EJ, Hayashi F, et al. Modulation of the synaptic drive to respiratory premotor and motor neurons. Respir Physiol 1997;110(2–3): 161–76.
13. Hajiha M, DuBord MA, Liu H, et al. Opioid receptor mechanisms at the hypoglossal motor pool and effects on tongue muscle activity in vivo. J Physiol 2009;587(Pt 11):2677–92.
14. Rekling JC, Funk GD, Bayliss DA, et al. Synaptic control of motoneuronal excitability. Physiol Rev 2000;80(2):767–852.
15. McKay LC, Feldman JL. Unilateral ablation of pre-botzinger complex disrupts breathing during sleep but not wakefulness. Am J Respir Crit Care Med 2008;178(1):89–95.
16. McKay LC, Janczewski WA, Feldman JL. Sleep-disordered breathing after targeted ablation of pre-Botzinger complex neurons. Nat Neurosci 2005; 8(9):1142–4.
17. Dahan A, van der Schrier R, Smith T, et al. Averting opioid-induced respiratory depression without affecting analgesia. Anesthesiology 2018;128(5): 1027–37.
18. Stucke AG, Levitt ES, Montandon G. Editorial: opioid-induced respiratory depression: neural circuits and cellular pathways. Front Physiol 2023; 14:1348910. https://doi.org/10.3389/fphys.2023.1348910.
19. Dick TE, Parmeggiani PL, Orem J. Intercostal muscle activity during sleep in the cat: an augmentation of expiratory activity. Respir Physiol 1982; 50(2):255–65.
20. Pisanski A, Pagliardini S. The parafacial respiratory group and the control of active expiration. Respir Physiol Neurobiol 2019;265:153–60.
21. Saini JK, Janes TA, MacLean JE, et al. Expiratory activity during sleep in children. J Sleep Res 2022; 31(4):e13539. https://doi.org/10.1111/jsr.13539.
22. Orem J, Dick T. Consistency and signal strength of respiratory neuronal activity. J Neurophysiol 1983; 50(5):1098–107.
23. Orem J, Osorio I, Brooks E, et al. Activity of respiratory neurons during NREM sleep. J Neurophysiol 1985;54(5):1144–56.
24. Horner RL. Respiratory physiology: central neural control of respiratory neurons and motoneurons during sleep. In: Kryger MH, Roth T, Goldstein CA, et al, editors. Principles and practice of sleep medicine. 7th edition. Philadelphia (PA): Elsevier; 2022. p. 233–44.
25. Orem J. Respiratory neurons and sleep. In: Kryger MH, Roth T, Dement WC, editors. Principles and practice of sleep medicine. 2nd edition. Philadelphia (PA): Saunders; 1994. p. 177–93.
26. Orem J, Lovering AT, Dunin-Barkowski W, et al. Tonic activity in the respiratory system in wakefulness, NREM and REM sleep. Sleep 2002;25(5):488–96.
27. Horner RL. Neural control of the upper airway: integrative physiological mechanisms and relevance for sleep disordered breathing. Compr Physiol 2012;2:479–535.
28. Henke KG, Badr MS, Skatrud JB, et al. Load compensation and respiratory muscle function during sleep. J Appl Physiol 1992;72(4):1221–34.
29. Hudgel DW, Martin RJ, Johnson B, et al. Mechanics of the respiratory system and breathing pattern during sleep in normal humans. J Appl Physiol 1984;56(1):133–7.
30. Hudgel DW, Devadatta P. Decrease in functional residual capacity during sleep in normal humans. J Appl Physiol 1984;57(5):1319–22.
31. Dempsey JA, Veasey SC, Morgan BJ, et al. Pathophysiology of sleep apnea. Physiol Rev 2010;90(1): 47–112. doi:90/1/47 [pii].
32. Goldstein RS. Hypoventilation: neuromuscular and chest wall disorders. Clin Chest Med 1992;13(3): 507–21.
33. Stradling JR, Kozar LF, Dark J, et al. Effect of acute diaphragm paralysis on ventilation in awake and sleeping dogs. Am Rev Respir Dis 1987;136(3): 633–7.
34. Bennett JR, Dunroy HM, Corfield DR, et al. Respiratory muscle activity during REM sleep in patients with diaphragm paralysis. Neurology 2004;62(1): 134–7.
35. Fink BR. The stimulant effect of wakefulness on respiration: clinical aspects. Br J Anaesth 1961; 33:97–101.
36. Orem J. The nature of the wakefulness stimulus for breathing. Prog Clin Biol Res 1990;345:23–30 [discussion: 31].
37. Phillipson EA, Bowes G. Control of breathing during sleep. In: Cherniack NS, Widdicombe JG, editors. Handbook of physiology, section 3, the respiratory system, vol II, control of breathing, part 2. Bethesda (MD): American Physiological Society; 1986. p. 649–89.
38. Duffin J, Mohan RM, Vasiliou P, et al. A model of the chemoreflex control of breathing in humans: model parameters measurement. Respir Physiol 2000; 120(1):13–26.
39. Dejours P. Chemoreflexes in breathing. Physiol Rev 1962;42:335–58.
40. Naughton M, Benard D, Tam A, et al. Role of hyperventilation in the pathogenesis of central sleep apneas in patients with congestive heart failure. Am Rev Respir Dis 1993;148(2):330–8.
41. Cardani S, Janes TA, Betzner W, et al. Knockdown of PHOX2B in the retrotrapezoid nucleus reduces

the central CO(2) chemoreflex in rats. eLife 2024; 13doi. https://doi.org/10.7554/eLife.94653.
42. Dubreuil V, Ramanantsoa N, Trochet D, et al. A human mutation in Phox2b causes lack of CO2 chemosensitivity, fatal central apnea, and specific loss of parafacial neurons. Proc Natl Acad Sci USA 2008;105(3):1067–72. doi:0709115105 [pii].
43. Weese-Mayer DE, Berry-Kravis EM. Genetics of congenital central hypoventilation syndrome: lessons from a seemingly orphan disease. Am J Respir Crit Care Med 2004;170(1):16–21.
44. Antic NA, Malow BA, Lange N, et al. PHOX2B mutation-confirmed congenital central hypoventilation syndrome: presentation in adulthood. Am J Respir Crit Care Med 2006;174(8):923–7.
45. Shea SA. Life without ventilatory chemosensitivity. Respir Physiol 1997;110(2–3):199–210.
46. Berry-Kravis EM, Zhou L, Rand CM, et al. Congenital central hypoventilation syndrome: PHOX2B mutations and phenotype. Am J Respir Crit Care Med 2006;174(10):1139–44.
47. Guyenet PG, Stornetta RL, Bayliss DA, et al. Retrotrapezoid nucleus: a litmus test for the identification of central chemoreceptors. Exp Physiol 2005;90(3): 247–53 [discussion: 253–7]. doi:expphysiol.2004.029637 [pii].
48. Mulkey DK, Stornetta RL, Weston MC, et al. Respiratory control by ventral surface chemoreceptor neurons in rats. Nat Neurosci 2004;7(12):1360–9.
49. Mitchell GS. Back to the future: carbon dioxide chemoreceptors in the mammalian brain. Nat Neurosci 2004;7(12):1288–90.
50. Richerson GB, Wang W, Hodges MR, et al. Homing in on the specific phenotype(s) of central respiratory chemoreceptors. Exp Physiol 2005;90(3): 259–66 [discussion: 266–9]. doi:expphysiol.2005.029843 [pii].
51. Foote SL, Bloom FE, Aston-Jones G. Nucleus locus ceruleus: new evidence of anatomical and physiological specificity. Phys Rev 1983;63(3): 844–914.
52. Jacobs BL, Fornal CA. 5-HT and motor control: a hypothesis. Trends Neurosci 1993;16(9):346–52.
53. Veasey SC, Fornal CA, Metzler CW, et al. Single-unit responses of serotonergic dorsal raphe neurons to specific motor challenges in freely moving cats. Neuroscience 1997;79(1):161–9.
54. Veasey SC, Fornal CA, Metzler CW, et al. Response of serotonergic caudal raphe neurons in relation to specific motor activities in freely moving cats. J Neurosci 1995;15(7 Pt 2):5346–59.
55. Buchanan GF, Richerson GB. Central serotonin neurons are required for arousal to CO2. Proc Natl Acad Sci USA 2010;107(37):16354–9. doi: 1004587107 [pii].
56. Nattie E, Li A. Central chemoreception is a complex system function that involves multiple brain stem sites. J Appl Physiol 2009;106(4):1464–6. doi:00112.2008 [pii].
57. Nattie EE. Central chemosensitivity, sleep, and wakefulness. Respir Physiol 2001;129(1–2):257–68. doi: S003456870100295X [pii].
58. Phillipson EA, Sullivan CE. Arousal: the forgotten response to respiratory stimuli. Am Rev Respir Dis 1978;118(5):807–9.
59. Douglas NJ, White DP, Weil JV, et al. Hypercapnic ventilatory response in sleeping adults. Am Rev Respir Dis 1982;126(5):758–62.
60. Caruana-Montaldo B, Gleeson K, Zwillich CW. The control of breathing in clinical practice. Chest 2000;117(1):205–25.
61. Lahiri S, Mokashi A, Mulligan E, et al. Comparison of aortic and carotid chemoreceptor responses to hypercapnia and hypoxia. J Appl Physiol Respir Environ Exerc Physiol 1981;51(1):55–61.
62. Lahiri S, Roy A, Baby SM, et al. Oxygen sensing in the body. Prog Biophys Mol Biol 2006;91(3): 249–86.
63. Nielsen M, Smith H. Studies on the regulation of respiration in acute hypoxia; with a appendix on respiratory control during prolonged hypoxia. Acta Physiol Scand 1952;24(4):293–313.
64. Prabhakar NR. O2 sensing at the mammalian carotid body: why multiple O2 sensors and multiple transmitters? Exp Physiol 2006;91(1):17–23.
65. Zhong H, Zhang M, Nurse CA. Synapse formation and hypoxic signalling in co-cultures of rat petrosal neurones and carotid body type 1 cells. J Physiol 1997;503(Pt 3):599–612.
66. Campanucci VA, Nurse CA. Autonomic innervation of the carotid body: role in efferent inhibition. Respir Physiol Neurobiol 2007;157(1):83–92. doi: S1569-9048(07)00037-7 [pii].
67. Lahiri S, Forster RE 2nd. CO2/H(+) sensing: peripheral and central chemoreception. Int J Biochem Cell Biol 2003;35(10):1413–35. doi:S1357272503000505 [pii].
68. Cotten JF, Keshavaprasad B, Laster MJ, et al. The ventilatory stimulant doxapram inhibits TASK tandem pore (K2P) potassium channel function but does not affect minimum alveolar anesthetic concentration. Anesth Analg 2006;102(3):779–85.
69. Schmickl CN, Landry S, Orr JE, et al. Effects of acetazolamide on control of breathing in sleep apnea patients: mechanistic insights using meta-analyses and physiological model simulations. Physiol Rep 2021;9(20):e15071. https://doi.org/10.14814/phy2.15071.
70. Douglas NJ, White DP, Weil JV, et al. Hypoxic ventilatory response decreases during sleep in normal men. Am Rev Respir Dis 1982;125(3):286–9.
71. Douglas NJ. Respiratory physiology: understanding the control of ventilation. In: Kryger MH, Roth T, Dement WC, editors. Principles and practice of

sleep medicine. 5th edition. Philadelphia (PA): Elsevier Saunders; 2011. p. 250–8.
72. Hunt CE, Hauck FR. Sudden infant death syndrome. CMAJ (Can Med Assoc J) 2006;174(13): 1861–9. doi:174/13/1861 [pii].
73. Eckert DJ, Younes MK. Arousal from sleep: implications for obstructive sleep apnea pathogenesis and treatment. J Appl Physiol 2014;116(3):302–13.
74. Kaur S, Pedersen NP, Yokota S, et al. Glutamatergic signaling from the parabrachial nucleus plays a critical role in hypercapnic arousal. J Neurosci 2013;33(18):7627–40.
75. Yokota S, Kaur S, VanderHorst VG, et al. Respiratory-related outputs of glutamatergic, hypercapnia-responsive parabrachial neurons in mice. J Comp Neurol 2015;523(6):907–20.
76. Kaur S, Wang JL, Ferrari L, et al. A genetically defined circuit for arousal from sleep during hypercapnia. Neuron 2017;96(5):1153–67.e5.
77. Kaur S, Saper CB. Neural circuitry underlying waking up to hypercapnia. Front Neurosci 2019; 13:401.
78. Kaur S, De Luca R, Khanday MA, et al. Role of serotonergic dorsal raphe neurons in hypercapnia-induced arousals. Nat Commun 2020;11(1):2769.
79. Gargaglioni LH, Hartzler LK, Putnam RW. The locus coeruleus and central chemosensitivity. Respir Physiol Neurobiol 2010;173(3):264–73. doi:S1569-9048(10)00160-6 [pii].
80. Hodges MR, Richerson GB. Medullary serotonin neurons and their roles in central respiratory chemoreception. Respir Physiol Neurobiol 2010;173(3): 256–63.
81. Abbott SBG, Souza G. Chemoreceptor mechanisms regulating CO2 -induced arousal from sleep. J Physiol 2021;599(10):2559–71.
82. Brown EN, Lydic R, Schiff ND. General anesthesia, sleep, and coma. N Engl J Med 2010;363(27): 2638–50.
83. Franks NP. General anaesthesia: from molecular targets to neuronal pathways of sleep and arousal. Nat Rev Neurosci 2008;9(5):370–86. doi:nrn2372 [pii].
84. Franks NP, Zecharia AY. Sleep and general anesthesia. Can J Anaesth 2011;58:139–48. Le sommeil et l'anesthesie generale.
85. Lydic R, Baghdoyan HA. Sleep, anesthesiology, and the neurobiology of arousal state control. Anesthesiology 2005;103(6):1268–95.
86. Orser BA. Extrasynaptic GABAA receptors are critical targets for sedative-hypnotic drugs. J Clin Sleep Med 2006;2(2):S12–8.
87. Belelli D, Lambert JJ. Neurosteroids: endogenous regulators of the GABA(A) receptor. Nat Rev Neurosci 2005;6(7):565–75. nrn1703 [pii].
88. Zhan G, Serrano F, Fenik P, et al. NADPH oxidase mediates hypersomnolence and brain oxidative injury in a murine model of sleep apnea. Am J Respir Crit Care Med 2005;172(7):921–9.
89. Kinney HC, Thach BT. The sudden infant death syndrome. N Engl J Med 2009;361(8):795–805. doi:361/8/795 [pii].
90. White DP, Younes MK. Obstructive sleep apnea. Compr Physiol 2012;2(4):2541–94.
91. Hedner J, Stenlof K, Zou D, et al. A randomized controlled clinical trial exploring safety and tolerability of sulthiame in sleep apnea. Am J Respir Crit Care Med 2022;205(12):1461–9.
92. Hoff E, Strassberger C, Zou D, et al. Modification of endotypic traits in OSA by the carbonic anhydrase inhibitor sulthiame. Chest 2024;165(3):704–15.
93. Eckert DJ, White DP, Jordan AS, et al. Defining phenotypic causes of obstructive sleep apnea. Identification of novel therapeutic targets. Am J Respir Crit Care Med 2013;188(8):996–1004.
94. Orr JE, Malhotra A, Sands SA. Pathogenesis of central and complex sleep apnoea. Respirology 2017;22(1):43–52.
95. Younes M, Ostrowski M, Thompson W, et al. Chemical control stability in patients with obstructive sleep apnea. Am J Respir Crit Care Med 2001; 163(5):1181–90.
96. Edwards BA, Sands SA, Eckert DJ, et al. Acetazolamide improves loop gain but not the other physiological traits causing obstructive sleep apnoea. J Physiol 2012;590(5):1199–211.
97. Wellman A, Eckert DJ, Jordan AS, et al. A method for measuring and modeling the physiological traits causing obstructive sleep apnea. J Appl Physiol 2011;110(6):1627–37.
98. Younes M. Role of respiratory control mechanisms in the pathogenesis of obstructive sleep disorders. J Appl Physiol 2008;105(5):1389–405.
99. Younes M, Loewen AH, Ostrowski M, et al. Genioglossus activity available via non-arousal mechanisms vs. that required for opening the airway in obstructive apnea patients. J Appl Physiol 2012; 112(2):249–58.
100. Younes M. Contributions of upper airway mechanics and control mechanisms to severity of obstructive apnea. Am J Respir Crit Care Med 2003;168: 645–58.
101. Malhotra A, Grunstein RR, Fietze I, et al. Tirzepatide for the treatment of obstructive sleep apnea and obesity. N Engl J Med 2024;391(13):1193–205.
102. Taranto-Montemurro L, Messineo L, Wellman A. Targeting endotypic traits with medications for the pharmacological treatment of obstructive sleep apnea. A review of the current literature. J Clin Med 2019;8(11):1846.
103. Messineo L, Sands SA, Labarca G. Hypnotics on obstructive sleep apnea severity and endotypes: a systematic review and meta-analysis. Am J Respir Crit Care Med 2024;210(12):1461–74.

Central Sleep Apnea
Pathophysiology, Diagnosis and Classification

Clodagh M. Ryan, MBBCh, BAO, MD, FRCPC[a,b,*], T. Douglas Bradley, MD[a,b]

KEYWORDS

• Central sleep apnea • Cheyne-Stokes respiration • Respiratory inductance plethysmography • Photoplethysmography • Loop gain • Chemosensitivity

KEY POINTS

- Central sleep apnea (CSA) is characterized by diminished airflow with reduced or absent respiratory effort. It is defined on the basis of polysomnographic (PSG) characteristics. In-laboratory PSG with dual belt respiratory inductance plethysmography is necessary to determine both effort and thoracoabdominal phase relationships. Some newer technologies such as photoplethysmography may serve a role in screening for CSA.
- CSA is a heterogenous disorder, and clinical classification is usually based on the presence or absence of hypercapnia.
- The pathophysiology of CSA is usually due to inadequate generation or transmission of the fundamental respiratory rhythm or ventilatory control instability. The engineering concept of loop gain is used to provide a quantitative framework to understand the instability within the ventilatory system.
- Nonhypercapnic CSA has a hyperresponsive ventilatory system that predisposes to cycles of hyperventilation that drive the Pa_{CO_2} below a level to maintain respiration, this level is referred to as the apneic threshold. It is associated with normocapnia or hypocapnia and is most prominent during nonrapid eye movement sleep. It is often characterized by a periodic (waxing and waning) pattern of respiration.
- Hypercapnic CSA is due to insufficient ventilatory output or failure of the neuromuscular apparatus. It is associated with sustained hypoventilation and CSA. It is most prominent during rapid eye movement sleep.

INTRODUCTION

Central sleep apnea (CSA) is a sleep breathing disorder (SBD) in which a transient reduction in respiratory drive leads to a corresponding reduction in airflow. This occurs repetitively throughout the night. It is a heterogenous disorder in which the pathophysiological mechanisms have not been fully elucidated due to the complex nature of the control of breathing (see Richard L. Horner's article, "Control of Breathing," in this issue). The absence of a clear understanding of the pathophysiological mechanisms underlying CSA and the need to better characterize and diagnosis CSA have been identified as necessary research priorities by the American Thoracic Society.[1] It is a relatively rare disorder occurring in less than 1% of the general population and is associated with cardiovascular, central nervous system, systemic, and genetic disorders. In this article, we will review the definition, diagnostic modalities, and classification of CSA and provide an overview of the pathophysiology.

[a] Division of Respirology, Department of Medicine, University of Toronto, Toronto, Ontario, Canada; [b] Sleep Research Laboratory, KITE Research Institute, University Health Network, Toronto, Ontario, M5G2A2, Canada
* Corresponding author. Toronto General Hospital, 9N-967, 585 University Avenue, Toronto M5G2N2, Canada.
E-mail address: Clodagh.ryan@uhn.ca

Sleep Med Clin 21 (2026) 299–316
https://doi.org/10.1016/j.jsmc.2026.06.004

Abbreviations

AASM	American Academy of Sleep Medicine
AHI	apnea-hypopnea index
AI	artificial intelligence
CPC	cardiopulmonary coupling
CSA	central sleep apnea
CSR	Cheyne-Stokes respiration
EEG	electroencephalogram
eLFC	elevated low frequency coupling
EMG	electromyography
EMG	electromyogram
EOG	electrooculogram
FRC	functional residual capacity
HF	heart failure
HFC	high frequency coupling
HRV	heart rate variability
HSAT	home sleep apnea testing
ICSD	International Classification of Sleep Disorders
LFC	low frequency coupling
LG	loop gain
LV	left ventricle
ML	machine learning
NREM	nonrapid eye movement
Pco_2	partial pressure of carbon dioxide
$Paco_2$	arterial partial pressure of carbon dioxide
Pao_2	arterial partial pressure of oxygen
PAT	peripheral arterial tone
PE	piezoelectric
PPG	photoplethysmography
PSG	polysomnographic
PSG	polysomnogram
PVDF	polyvinylidene fluoride
REM	rapid eye movement
RIP	respiratory inductance plethysmography
SBD	sleep breathing disorder
SNA	sympathetic nervous system
SpO2	pulse oxygen saturation
VE	minute ventilation

CENTRAL SLEEP APNEA DEFINITION

CSA is defined based on polysomnographic (PSG) characteristics with subsequent classification formulated from the underlying etiology. According to the American Academy of Sleep Medicine (AASM), the PSG definition of a central apnea in adults is a reduction in airflow of $\geq$90% for $\geq$10 seconds in the absence of respiratory effort and of a central hypopnea, is a reduction in airflow of $\geq$ 30% to 90% from the baseline peak level $\geq$10 seconds in association with an oxygen desaturation or a cortical arousal in the absence of evidence of upper airway obstruction (ie, in-phase thoraco-abdominal motion on respiratory inductance plethysmography [RIP] without flattening of the nasal airflow signal).[2] The definition differs in children and is reviewed in Indra Narang and colleagues' article, "CSA and hypoventilation disorderes in children," in this issue. The differentiation from obstructive events is critical: events are scored as obstructive if there is any of the following: snoring, increased inspiratory flattening of the nasal airflow signal, and associated thoracoabdominal paradoxic motion on RIP during the event but not during pre-event breathing. CSA occurs primarily during nonrapid eye movement (NREM) sleep[3–6] in conditions associated with ventilatory instability (eg, heart failure [HF]), but are rapid eye movement (REM)-predominant in those with defects in the respiratory control system or neuromuscular apparatus,[7,8] except for opioid induced CSA. This is likely attributable to opioids elevating ventilatory instability through an augmentation in loop gain (LG) and respiratory rate variability as well as disruption of respiratory rhythm generation.[9,10] CSA is also more frequent in the supine position.[4,11,12] Other metrics described include the timing and profile of oxygen desaturation and resaturation (**Box 1**).

Thus, the differentiation between central and obstructive events is often challenging and most sleep centers choose not to delineate hypopneas as either central or obstructive or default to obstructive.[13] Since hypopneas are far more common than apneas, classification would be based on a minority of events which could lead to a significant underestimation of the prevalence of CSA because of misclassification as OSA with adverse impacts on treatment decisions.[14,15]

Box 1
Polysomnographic findings suggestive of central hypopneas

NREM-related events

No snoring during the hypopnea

No thoracoabdominal paradox during the hypopnea

Periodic breathing pattern with gradual event termination

Arousal at the peak of ventilation

SaO_2 Profile

- Nadir delayed due to prolonged circulation time
- Peak in the midst of the hypopnea
- Desaturation and resaturation in a periodic pattern
- Modest drop in the oxygen saturation

PATHOPHYSIOLOGY OF CENTRAL SLEEP APNEA

Central events are defined by the absence of respiratory effort, with a period of hyperpnea alternating with an apneic or hypopneic phase and are usually cyclical. They are caused by 2 major mechanisms, *the inadequate generation or transmission of the fundamental respiratory rhythm or ventilatory control instability*. These distinct mechanisms may cause hypercapnic or nonhypercapnic CSA, respectively. CSA due to ventilatory control instability is generally more common. In some instances, there may be dual processes with both dysregulation of ventilatory control and respiratory rhythm generation, for example, opioid-induced CSA.[10] Common to all forms of CSA is the reduction of the $Paco_2$ below a level to maintain respiration, and this level is referred to as the apneic threshold.

Sleep-Dependent Vulnerability: Effect of Sleep and Sleep-Wake Transition on Ventilatory Control

As discussed in the Richard L. Horner's article, "Control of Breathing," in this issue during normal breathing, there is a continuous tonic activity to the respiratory muscles from the central respiratory neurons located in the medulla oblongata and pons of the lower brainstem (behavioral control system). This activity is impacted by sleep with a differential effect dependent on the neurons and sleep state. A withdrawal of this excitatory drive to breathe at sleep onset results in a dependence on the metabolic control system which is derived predominantly from the central chemoreceptors (principally the arterial partial pressure of carbon dioxide ($Paco_2$)) with a small contribution from peripheral chemoreceptors[16] (**Fig. 1**). This serves to accentuate and unmask deficiencies within the cardiorespiratory system, control of breathing and neuromuscular apparatus. Under normal conditions on transition to sleep, there is a reduction in ventilation, and the eupneic CO2 ($PaCO_{2eupnea}$) rises by 2 to 4 mm Hg.[17] During this time even in healthy individuals, there are transient reductions in the $Paco_2$ below the apnea threshold ($PaCO_{2AT}$) for sleep—the level below which the pontomedullary respiratory rhythm generator stops firing.[18,19] This results in a loss of respiratory drive with a fall in ventilation and a central apnea ensues until the $Paco_2$ rises above the threshold level for rhythm generation in sleep, and breathing resumes. If consolidated sleep is achieved no further central events occur, but ongoing sleep-wake transitions can destabilize ventilation and is dependent on the difference between wake and sleep $Paco_2$ and the steepness of the ventilatory response to CO2 during wake.[20] This critical dependence on the metabolic control system persists during light NREM sleep making it vulnerable to transient increases in ventilation and ventilatory instability. In contrast during REM sleep, there is greater tonic excitatory input. For this reason, central events are more frequent during NREM sleep.[21] This contrasts to a REM predominance in those with defects in generation of respiratory rhythm when additional converging physiologic changes amplify vulnerabilities during this sleep state[8] (**Fig. 2**).

Nonhypercapnic Central Sleep Apnea—Ventilatory Control Instability

The fundamental cause of central apneas and hypopneas in *non.hypercapnic CSA* is a fall in $Paco_2$ toward (hypopnea) or below (apnea) the apneic threshold[6,22] This is demonstrated by the observation that raising $Paco_2$ above the apnea threshold via inhalation of CO2 or addition of dead-space instantaneously abolishes idiopathic CSA[23] and CSA-CSR in HF.[24] There are multiple factors contributing to the tendency to hyperventilate and drive $Paco_2$ below the apnea threshold.

Mathematical models have been developed to explain the instability within the respiratory control system and to provide an understanding of CSA, particularly that associated with Cheyne-Stokes respiration (CSR).[25,26] This uses control system engineering concepts to provide a quantitative framework for the propensity of ventilatory instability. Physiologic homeostasis is usually achieved through negative feedback. Based on this model, any perturbation in ventilation will elicit a response to maintain blood gas tensions (above and below eupnea), chiefly the $Paco_2$ within a narrow range which varies dependent on sleep state. Changes in blood gas tensions are sensed at the chemoreceptors, principally the peripheral (carotid bodies) rather than the central (medullary brain stem). Because the change in ventilation in response to a perturbation is not instantaneous, the inherent delays cause respiratory instability and ongoing oscillation of ventilation, due to the reduction in the $Paco_2$ below the apneic threshold.

LG quantifies the magnitude of the corrective ventilatory response relative to the disturbance. An LG greater than 1 represents an unstable ventilatory system (hyperresponsive) whereby the magnitude of the response is greater than the initial disturbance and the system over-shoots and under-shoots perpetuating the ventilatory disturbance. Therefore, trivial changes in blood

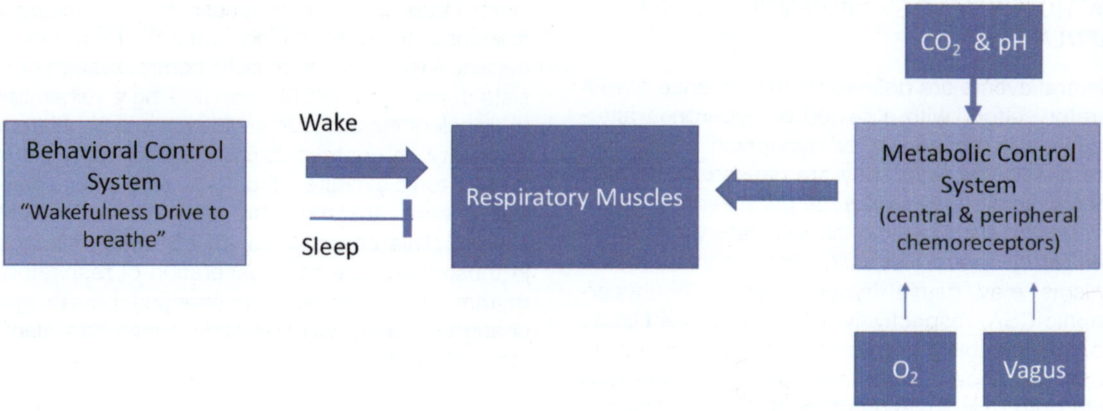

Fig. 1. Schematic of the respiratory control system. This is a simplified representation of the respiratory control system. The metabolic or automatic control system regulates gas homeostasis and acid-base balance through inputs from the peripheral (carotid bodies), central (medullary system) chemoreceptors, and the vagus nerve. The behavioral or voluntary control system is integrated within the brainstem automatic system and control volitional acts (eg, phonation) that require respiratory maneuvers.[123]

gas tensions may result in marked fluctuations in ventilation. This is manifest by increased respiratory responsiveness of the peripheral and central chemoreceptors, which predisposes to hyperventilation.[6,27] An LG less than 1 is deemed to be a more stable system but may lead to unstable breathing in certain circumstances.[28] The classic 3 components of LG include controller, plant,

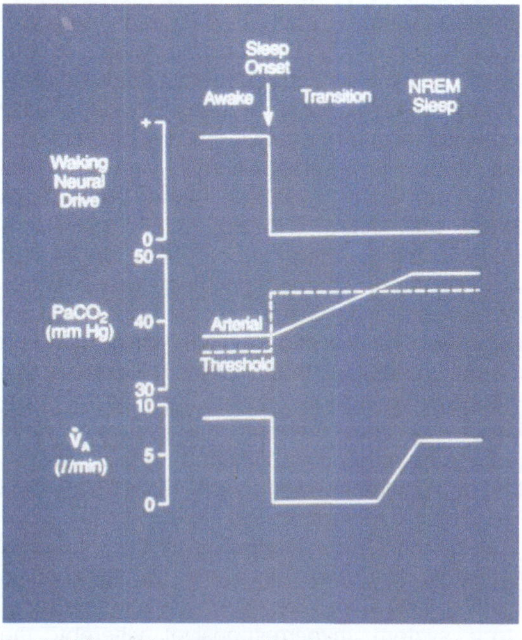

Fig. 2. Schematic diagram showing a proposed mechanism underlying central sleep apnea. $Paco_2$, partial pressure of carbon dioxide; REM, rapid eye movement; V, ventilation. (Created in BioRender. Ryan, C. (2026) https://BioRender.com/47qoyqy.)

and mixing gain. Each of these components may contribute to the propensity for ventilatory instability. LG is not static and varies both during sleep states (higher in NREM sleep than REM sleep) and over the course of the night.[29]

Controller gain represents the sensitivity of the chemoreceptors to changes in $Paco_2$ and Pao_2 $\left(\frac{\Delta VE}{PaCO2} / > <eupnea\right)$. The ventilatory response is amplified if there are increased chemosensitivity or oversensitive chemoreceptors.[20] *Plant gain* is the effectiveness of ventilation in altering blood gas tensions ($\Delta PaCO2 / \Delta VE$). This is influenced by reduced CO2 stores and functional residual capacity (FRC), increased dead space ventilation, baseline ventilation, metabolic CO2 production, and reduced cardiac output (which determines rate of CO2 delivery to the lung).[30,31] *Mixing gain* is a measure of the circulatory delay (lung-to-chemoreceptor delay) and the time taken to effect a change. A long circulation time delays the feedback to the system and prolongs oscillation time (**Fig. 3**).

Another important component in LG is the *CO2 reserve*, which is the difference between $Paco_2$ at eupnea and at the apnea threshold ($PaCO_{2eupnea}$ – $PaCO_{2AT}$). This varies inversely with plant gain and the slope of the ventilatory response to reduced CO2 below eupnea. In the presence of a narrow CO2 reserve, transient small changes in ventilation will more readily induce central apneas.[20] The CO2 reserve varies and is lower in men compared to women, and older adults compared to younger.[32,33]

There are several other contributory factors that may modulate LG and ventilatory stability.

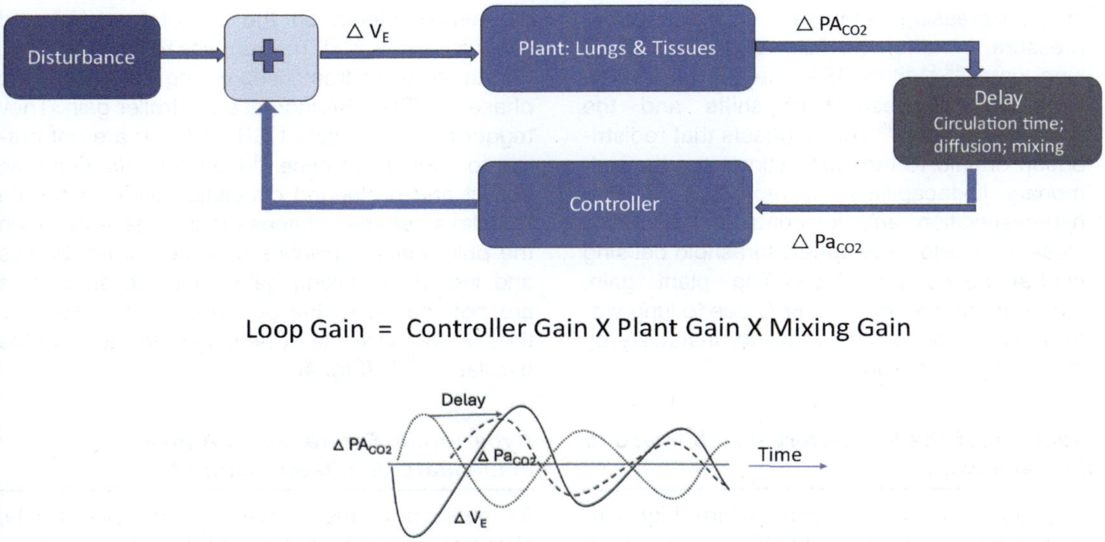

Fig. 3. A schematic diagram of the negative feedback control system controlling ventilation. A disturbance in breathing causes a reduction in ventilation and a drop in the arterial partial pressure of carbon dioxide ($Paco_2$) below the apnea threshold, followed by a cessation of breathing and subsequent rise in $Paco_2$. Controller gain reflects the sensitivity of the peripheral and central chemoreceptors to changes in blood gas tensions and determines the magnitude of the drive to the ventilatory muscles. Plant gain reflects the effectiveness of the lungs to change $Paco_2$. Mixing gain measures delays within the system. Loop gain (LG) is the product of controller, plant, and mixing gain. If LG is greater than 1, the oscillations in ventilation will increase in amplitude and self-perpetuate. P_{ACO2}, alveolar carbon dioxide; VE, minute ventilation.

1. Sleep-Related Arousals: These serve to transiently restore the wakefulness drive to breathe and the $Paco_2$ levels that were present during sleep are considered a hypercapnic stimulus during wakefulness, causing a surge in ventilation and a reduction in the $Paco_2$ below the apnea threshold upon transition back to sleep causing a central apnea. The arousals increase LG by raising controller gain. Factors such as the timing of the arousal (those occurring at the beginning of the hyperpneic phase) and the intensity of the arousals has been shown to be proportional to ventilatory overshoot and duration of the apnea.[21,34,35] Although arousals are amplifiers of central apneas, they are not required to trigger events.[34]
2. Upper Airway Changes: Upper airway narrowing may occur during central apneic events due to the withdrawal of central respiratory drive causing reduced activation of the upper airway muscle and predisposing to upper airway collapsibility. Collapse of the upper airway promotes possible ventilatory overshoot on termination of the apnea, causing further ventilatory instability.[36,37] Conversely, in CSA-CSR reduced upper airway resistance has been described, attributable to augmented ventilation because of rostral fluid shifts stimulating the pulmonary juxtacapillary receptors which likely increases upper airway dilator muscle activity.[38]
3. Reduced FRC: During sleep ventilation oscillates around the FRC, which is the volume of gas present in the lung during tidal breathing. The FRC represents the alveolar gas reservoir which is responsible for buffering fluctuations in the CO2 and oxygen.[39] When FRC is reduced, there is a smaller gas reservoir and even small changes in alveolar ventilation can produce larger swings in the CO2 alveolar fraction, leading to greater swings in the $Paco_2$ and potential reduction in the Pco_2 below the apneic threshold.[40,41] There is also reduced oxygen reservoir and a propensity for greater hypoxemia which will trigger the peripheral chemoreceptors leading to ventilatory overshoot and perpetuation of the cycle. Both supine position and pulmonary congestion reduce FRC and are associated with worsening of CSA.[3,42] Therefore, reduced FRC promotes CSA primarily through an increase in plant gain.
4. Rostral Fluid Shifts: Overnight rostral fluid shifts occur between the extravascular and intravascular spaces when going from the upright to recumbent position.[43] In fluid overloaded states with elevated venous pressure the volume of fluid movement is greater, and this fluid may redistribute from the legs to the heart and

lungs, increasing pulmonary capillary wedge pressure, intrathoracic fluid, and extracellular lung water.[42,44,45] In CSA, there is an inverse correlation between fluid shifts and the nocturnal P_{CO_2}.[38,46] This suggests that redistribution of fluid to the lungs stimulates the pulmonary juxtacapillary (J) receptors causing hyperventilation and lowering of the Pa_{CO_2} close to or below the apneic threshold causing central apnea and increasing plant gain. Furthermore, the reduced FRC due to lung water may compound the ventilator instability by increasing plant gain.

Integration of the Ventilatory Instability/Loop Gain Framework

In conditions such as HF, renal failure, high altitude, and treatment-emergent CSA, there is high LG predominantly because of elevated controller gain.[27] These conditions usually have normocapnia or hypocapnia. CSA due to neuromuscular, neuromuscular junction, brainstem, or spinal cord disorders may have elevated plant gain contributing to high LG with associated hypercapnia.[47–49] Some clinical conditions may have changes to both controller and plant gain. Below, we will provide an outline of the pathophysiology of HF to provide an overview of the how the LG framework and ventilatory instability promotes CSA.

HF one of the commonest causes of CSA is a prototypical high LG state with hyperresponsiveness due to chronic hyperventilation. There are several factors in HF that interact to cause this high LG. The primary pathophysiological mechanism contributing to CSR-CSA is augmented peripheral and central chemosensitivity to CO2 (controller gain) and a propensity to ventilatory overshoot.[27,30,50,51] The exact molecular mechanisms causing increased chemosensitivity are unknown. Proposed mechanism includes: (a) purinergic signaling and/or build-up of reactive oxidative species (due to the chronic sympathetic activation) in the carotid bodies, that lower the threshold for chemoreceptor firing[52] and (b) low carotid blood flow causing reduced shear stress and down-regulation of a transcription factor that mediates carotid body chemoreflex sensitivity.[53] Second, elevated left heart filling pressures cause fluid overload with pulmonary congestion and activation of the pulmonary juxtacapillary receptors that augment central drive and ventilation and increase plant gain.[54] This is potentiated by rostral fluid shifts and reductions in the FRC.[42] Third, the possible role of impaired cerebral vascular reactivity and blood flow responses to CO2 with differential effects on the cerebral arterial and venous vessels.[55,56] This remains to be confirmed. Fourth, arousals from sleep during the hyperpneic phase of CSR-CSA increase controller gain. They trigger and propagate CSR-CSA but are not critical to CSA occurrence.[34] Lastly, the low cardiac output and prolonged circulation time contribute to delays between changes in the Pa_{CO_2} between the pulmonary capillaries and the carotid bodies and increases mixing gain. While these factors are not crucial to the occurrence of CSR-CSA, they do increase the cycle length and amplify the oscillation[30,57] (**Fig. 4**).

Hypercapnic Central Sleep Apnea—Inadequate Ventilatory Output

As outlined in the Richard L. Horner's article, "Control of Breathing," in this issue, the automatic process of breathing originates from the central respiratory rhythm generator located in the pons and medulla. The pre-Botzinger complex generates the fundamental respiratory rhythm and conveys this rhythmic activity to the inspiratory neurons of the dorsal and ventral respiratory groups that drive input to spinal motoneurons responsible for the activation of respiratory muscles. Diseases that cause dysfunction, neuronal cell loss,[58] or outright defects[59] in the pre-Botzinger complex result in diminished respiratory drive. During wakefulness, the suppressed respiratory drive will manifest with some degree of hypercapnia. This becomes more apparent during sleep when the loss of the wakefulness drive to sleep is abolished and the stimulatory influence of behavioral, cortical, and reticular inputs to the brain-stem respiratory neurons are reduced such that breathing becomes critically dependent on the defective metabolic respiratory control system resulting in more pronounced hypercapnia during sleep than wakefulness.[60,61] Coincident with this reduction in ventilation, there is an elevation in the P_{CO_2}, a reduction in the Pa_{O_2}, and a markedly elevated P_{CO_2} apneic threshold. There is high LG because of the low lung volumes which cause elevation in plant gain. CSA is more frequent and severe during REM sleep than NREM due to partial paralysis of the respiratory muscles and further reductions in ventilation.[8] Impaired neuromuscular transmission or mechanical limitation may also result in hypercapnic CSA. The CSA manifests as hypoventilation with central apneas and hypopneas. These central events do not have the waxing and waning pattern of ventilation evident with CSA due to ventilatory instability.

In neurodegenerative diseases (such as Parkinson disease, amyotrophic lateral sclerosis, multiple

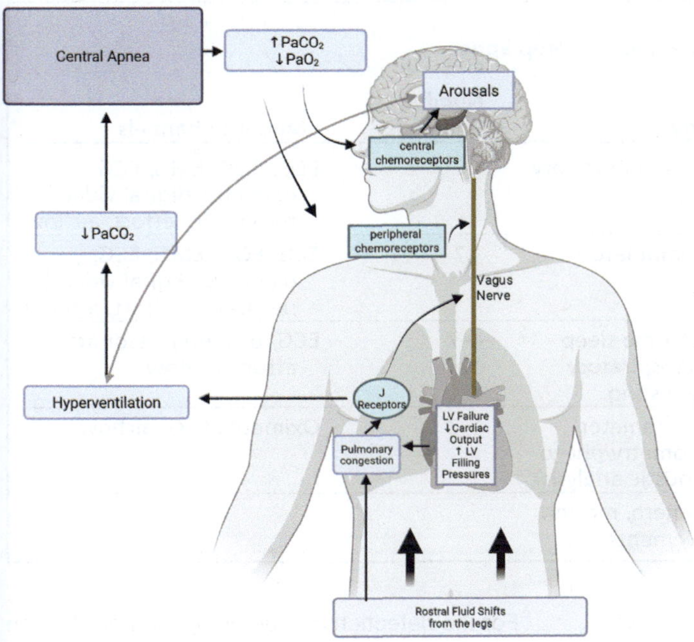

Fig. 4. Pathophysiology of central sleep apnea in heart failure (HF). J receptors, Juxtacapillary receptors. LV, left ventricle; $Paco_2$, arterial partial pressure of carbon dioxide; Pao_2, arterial partial pressure of oxygen. (Created in BioRender. Ryan C. 2026.)

system atrophy, or Leigh's syndrome), the development of CSA is proposed to be due to loss of neurons in the pre-Botzinger complex.[58] In multiple sclerosis, CSA is reported in those with medullary lesions affecting the respiratory neurons.[62]

Diseases affecting the brainstem, such as tumors, stroke, or Chiari malformation,[63] may cause CSA. Although, the central respiratory generator is predominantly in the medulla, there are projections to other areas of the brain and CSA may arise due to physical compression of the brainstem, stretching of the lower cranial nerves impeding those that carry inputs from the peripheral chemoreceptors, depletion of medullary chemosensitive neurons, or impact on the central pattern generator located in the dorsolateral pons.

Neuromuscular disorders (inherited and acquired myopathies) may result in hypoventilation and hypercapnic CSA. These diseases impair inspiratory muscle function including the diaphragm leading to alveolar hypoventilation. At the transition from wakefulness to sleep, the associated reduction in ventilatory response to CO2 and hypoxia, combined with the loss of respiratory muscle tone can lead to CSA.[64] While there is some central output to the respiratory muscles, strictly speaking, events may not be central, however, the muscles are unable to respond such that there is either markedly reduced or no muscle force generation leading events that appear central. Furthermore, on arousal from sleep, sleep position or state change small increases in ventilation may induce markedly exaggerated drops in the $Paco_2$ which is due to increased plant gain.

Medications that act on the inspiratory neurons in the pre-Botzinger complex can induce respiratory depression. These include opioids, baclofen, and valproic acid.[65] Opioids act via mu-opioid receptors which are expressed throughout the brainstem. The effect on respiratory neurons is dose-dependent and region specific. Opioids suppress the medullary pre-Botzinger complex[66] and the pontine Kolliker-Fuse nucleus causing respiratory depression and ataxic breathing.[67] They also have a differential effect inhibiting the firing of inspiratory rather than expiratory neurons.[68] In addition to the inhibition of rhythm generation, chronic opioids also cause ventilatory instability through heightened peripheral chemosensitivity with blunted central chemosensitivity (high LG) and a narrow CO2 reserve.[10,65,69] The CSA pattern in opioids may be a distinctive ataxic pattern, but a periodic pattern has also been described.[70] CSA may be hypercapnic or nonhypercapnic in opioid users dependent on the predominant underlying pathophysiological mechanisms.

TECHNIQUES FOR DIAGNOSING CENTRAL SLEEP APNEA

Diagnostic modalities for the determination of SBDs are classified into type 1 to 4 devices[71,72] (**Table 1**). In-laboratory polysomnogram (PSG) is

Table 1
Classification of diagnostic testing modalities for sleep apnea

Device Type	Description/Terminology	Number of Channels	Standard Channels
Type 1	Full technician-attended in-laboratory polysomnogram (PSG)	≥7	EEG, EOG, EMG, ECG, oximetry, digital video, respiratory effort, airflow
Type 2	Full unattended PSG—ambulatory	≥7	EEG, EOG, EMG, ECG, oximetry, digital video, respiratory effort, airflow
Type 3	Limited channel device/home sleep apnea testing (HSAT)/respiratory polygraphy, portable testing	4–7	ECG, oximetry, respiratory effort, airflow
Type 4	Oximetry and another parameter (eg, pulse arterial tonometry/photo-plethysmography, acoustic analysis)	1–2	Oximetry, ECG, airflow
Noncontact sensor	Acoustic analysis, 3D camera, motion sensors for micromovements		

the traditional gold standard test, however, with increased comorbid longevity in Western world populations and a need to provide SBD testing to greater numbers within health care systems buckling under financial, personnel, and bed resource constraints. Type 3 testing (limited channel/home sleep apnea testing) is often the routine testing modality. There are no universal technical standards for these devices[73] although it is recommended that a minimum of 3 sensors is necessary to provide the physiologic data to diagnose SBD.[74] Emerging newer technologies and wearables that harness artificial intelligence (AI) diagnose SBD through surrogate markers of autonomic function or through nonintrusive assessments of body movements, breathing, voice, and sound patterns. Currently, these limited channel (home sleep apnea testing [HSAT]) diagnostic testing modalities are recommended for those with a high pretest probability of SDB,[73] primarily OSA.[75] Validation studies of limited channel devices in those with CSA are infrequent and the wholesale use of this technology within the general population will likely lead to further misdiagnosis or misclassification of SDB in some patients. HSAT devices have limited regulatory approval for CSA detection dependent on jurisdiction. There have been small HSAT studies demonstrating high diagnostic accuracy (84%–91.4%) for CSA.[76–78] A more recent study by Tung and colleagues, evaluated the automated scoring algorithms on HSAT showing that there was systematic misclassification of central apneas as obstructive, producing erroneous assessment of CSA, and while manual scoring was superior, there were significant differences from PSG results.[79]

For the detection and determination of CSA, an assessment of respiratory effort or an inference of its absence from surrogate physiologic signals, is required in association with reduced airflow.[2] This absence of respiratory effort is the defining feature that differentiates central from obstructive events. Recent guidelines continue to recommend in-laboratory PSG for the accurate determination of CSA.[80] Therefore, in specific populations (eg, HF, atrial fibrillation, renal failure, neuromuscular disorders, neurologic disorders, on medications such as opioids) limited channel testing should be avoided.

Signal Modalities for the Detection of Central Sleep Apnea

As previously outlined, the ability to determine the presence of reduced or absence respiratory effort is a key to the detection of a central events. The "gold standard" is considered the direct measurement of intrathoracic pressure performed with an esophageal pressure catheter which accurately detects changes in respiratory effort. On inspiration, the pressure recordings are more negative than on expiration. However, during central events negative esophageal pressure is reduced (hypopnea) or absent (apnea), in contrast to obstructive events, in which inspiratory negative pressure swings are increased reflecting continuing respiratory drive against the occluded upper airway.[81] It is infrequently used in the clinical setting and usually limited to the research or critical care setting due to the invasive nature of the test. Alternative modalities include respitrace inductance plethysmography (RIP), photoplethysmography (PPG), cardiopulmonary coupling (CPC), seismocardiography, chest accelerometry ,and capacitive respiratory effort sensing to name a few. Testing for CSA detection has not been performed for many of these technologies (**Table 2**).

Respiratory inductance plethysmography

Measurement of respiratory motion, which reflects respiratory effort is routinely assessed by RIP.[2] RIP consists of 2 elastic bands within which are embedded insulated wire coils: one thoracic band positioned around the ribcage and the second positioned around the abdominal. The output is a thorax and abdominal signal and tidal volume signal which is the electronic sum of the 2 bands. Changes in the belts cross-sectional area during inspiration and expiration generate a digital signal proportional to the change in area. Although this is often referred to as a measure of effort, strictly speaking it is not since it does not measure pressure: rather, it is a measure of respiratory motion. This provides a semiquantitative assessment of inspiratory movement and estimate relative changes in tidal volume and ventilation in sleep apnea.[82] Calibration of RIP can be performed to estimate absolute tidal volume or flow. This is usually not performed in clinical practice and belt slippage; signal drift and positional changes can impact the volume estimates.[83,84] The design and quality of the RIP belts is important as it can affect the reliability and quality of the signals.[85,86]

Dual belt RIP technology is necessary to determine both effort and thoracoabdominal phase relationships. This is critical to differentiate between central and obstructive events. In central apneas, there is no excursion of the thoracoabdominal belts but in obstructive apneas there is reduced excursion and asynchronous motion. More recently, AI and machine learning (ML) signal processing methods have been explored to extract additional information from RIP including quantification of advanced ventilation metrics (% reduction in ventilation X duration X rate) and detection of arousals and sleep for obstructive sleep apnea.[87,88] AI/ML RIP algorithms have the potential to improve raw RIP and improve the differentiation between obstructive and central events.[89]

RIP in CSA can also be informative for guiding potential underlying etiology. In CSR-CSA, RIP Sum shows a characteristic crescendo-decrescendo pattern, whereas in opioid-induced CSA there may be an irregular ataxic or biot's pattern. In high-altitude CSA, the cycle length (apnea and hyperpnea duration) of events is short (15–20 seconds) with regular cycles.

While RIP is the preferred technology to assess respiratory effort, other methods including strain gauges, piezoelectric (PE) sensors, impedance plethysmography, and polyvinylidene fluoride (PVDF). PE belts have a single sensor which measures stretch or tension.[90] PVDF is a PE polymer which creates an electric charge when stretched and is used in PE belts. PVDF are considered acceptable for measurement of effort but have limited validation particularly for central events.[91,92]

Photoplethysmography

PPG is the technology embedded within a number of HSAT devices and consumer wearables. It is derived from a noninvasive optical technique with light emitting photodiode sensors that detect red (λ = 660 nm) and infrared (λ = 850–940 nm) light, and more recently green wavelength (λ = 530 nm) is included particularly in wearables. The sensors are placed on the forehead, wrist, or fingertip. Pulsatile changes in blood volume in the microvascular bed are detected. The waveform has an AC and DC component. The AC component tracks arterial pulsation and the DC reflects vasomotor and respiratory modulations.[93] Importantly, PPG does not measure respiratory effort and respiratory events are inferred from 3 respiratory-linked components

Table 2
Signal modalities for the detection of central sleep apnea

Signal Modality	Effort Detection	CSA/OSA Discrimination	Evidence Quality
Esophageal pressure	Direct	Yes (definitive)	Gold standard
Dual RIP	Direct	Yes (phase angle)	Strong
PPG (PAT)+ accelerometry	Indirect	Limited	Low/moderate
PPG-only	Indirect	Promising	Early
PPG + oximetry	Indirect	Promising	Early
CPC	Indirect	Yes	Moderate (ECG) Weak (PPG)
3D Time of Flight camera	Indirect	Possible	None
Mattress technologies	Indirect	Possible	None

that modulate the PPG signal. These include assessment of changes in amplitude, heart rate variability (HRV) and vasomotor changes. PPG amplitude oscillation occurs due to changes in intrathoracic pressure during respiration which alters cardiac venous return and stroke volume. This feature is extracted to represent respiratory effort derived respiration (PPGDR). HRV is extracted from the pulse to pulse interval from the PPG signal which mirrors the RR interval from the ECG. During apneic events surges in the pulse rate align with sympathetic nervous system (SNA) activation. Lastly, the vasomotor changes (ie, peripheral vasoconstriction) due to the increased SNA near the termination of apneic events are evident by acute drop in pulse wave amplitude on the PPG. This peripheral arterial tone (PAT) signal is used in some HSAT devices.

The discrimination between central and obstructive events on PPG is based on the fundamental difference in amplitude variation. The persistent ineffective respiratory effort during obstructive events generates high negative intrathoracic pressures and greater amplitude variation on the PPG signal. In contrast, central events due to the absence of effort are represented by flattening of the PPG amplitude signal.

Few studies have evaluated PPG algorithms for CSA classification.[94–97] A key prospective multicenter study by Massie and colleagues, studied 266 subjects who underwent parallel in-laboratory PSG and PPG on the finger-tip using the NightOwl device.[95] Of the subjects studied, 8.6% and 10.3% had central AHI (cAHI) greater than 10 and greater than 5 events per hour, respectively. The PPG signal processing included respiratory event analysis through SpO2 drops, pulse rate surges, and PAT signal changes. Subsequently, there were a further 5 steps which included filtering of the signal with retention of respiratory modulation, further extraction and normalization of the PPGDR signal, feature extraction applied to each PPGDR, signal quality rejection, ensemble of tree classifier and lastly cAHI extrapolation. For cAHI $\geq$ 10, the accuracy was 97.6%, with a high LR of 90.7 and low LR of 0.19. Notable limitations of the study include the small numbers, limited demographics, and uncertain generalizability. This CSA classifier was superior on benchmark comparison to the Pillar and colleagues, WatchPAT study which used PPG and accelerometry and had a lower sensitivity (cAHI $\geq$ 10, sensitivity 71.4% vs 81%).[96] Lazazzera and colleagues evaluated PPG with pulse oximetry and while the accuracy for detection of central compared to obstructive apnea and hypopneas was high (92.6% and 83.7%, respectively), the overall accuracy for detection of events (total apnea-hypopnea index [AHI]) was lower at 75.1%.[94] Lastly, an earlier small study in 2012, of Morpheus Ox, demonstrated sensitivity for the detection of central events of 82%.[97]

Presently, PPG is not recommended for the diagnosis of CSA, but may have a role in future CSA screening or to be incorporated within in-laboratory PSGs. Future larger, longitudinal and multi-night studies are required. CSA subtypes (opioid induced, high-altitude) have not been validated and characterization of the waxing and waning pattern of CSR has not been modeled. Confounders for PPG reliability and signal quality include atrial fibrillation, peripheral vasoconstriction, low cardiac output, and overnight fluid shifts.

Cardiopulmonary coupling

This is a signal-processing methodology which utilizes the known entrainment of heart rate to respiration. In NREM sleep due to a shift to increased parasympathetic tone, the synchronization of the heart rate with respiration (ie, respiratory sinus arrhythmia) is most pronounced.[98] This is quantified in CPC as high frequency coupling (HFC) occurring in the 0.1–0.4 Hz spectral band.[99] In REM sleep and wake periods, there is very low frequency coupling (LFC) below 0.01 Hz. Lastly, during periods of sleep fragmentation, or apnea when there is more sympathetic activation with fluctuations in heart rate and tidal volume, there is LFC between 0.01 and 0.1 Hz.[100]

The CPC algorithm is extracted from a single lead electrocardiogram ECG or PPG. The signals extracted are (a) normal to normal interval series from the R waves and (b) ECG-derived respiration or PPG amplitude modulation as a surrogate for the respiratory signal. Following extraction, the signals are resampled using cubic splines at 2 Hz, spectral analysis is performed with a derived measure of cardio-respiratory oscillatory power as a function of frequency and time. This is the CPC spectrogram.[101] The logarithm of the HFC/LFC is a summary metric, with low values representing unstable or apnea-related sleep.[102] Within the LFC zone, further analysis identifies an elevated LFC (eLFC) with a narrow band (NB) (0.006–0.1 Hz) and broad band (BB) (0.01–0.1 Hz). The $eLFC_{NB}$ correlates to central/complex apnea, periodic breathing or high LG states, and the $eLFC_{BB}$ correlates with obstructive sleep apnea.[103] Overall, CPC $eLFC_{NB}$ has modest correlation with PSG central event scoring (r = 0.18; $P<.001$) and the presence of cardiac arrhythmias (ECG-based CPC) or peripheral vasoconstriction (PPG-based CPC) impedes the reliability of CPC. It may have a role in improving diagnostic accuracy in conjunction with traditional RIP technologies.

Other technologies

Mattress technologies use noncontact mechanical (eg, ballistocardiography), radar, radiofrequency identification, or optical sensors in combination with sound data to detect surrogates of cardiopulmonary activity and sleep, with the use of ML to estimate the AHI. Although, many of the devices have high diagnostic accuracy for moderate to severe sleep apnea, there are no validation studies for the discrimination between obstructive and central events.[104] The relatively low prevalence of CSA limits the power to design, train, and validate for central events in datasets. Although there is not a separate assessment of thoracic versus abdominal effort necessary for the determination of central events, investigators have indicated that CSA event determination is feasible due to the distinct lack of movement noted on visual inspection of the signals.[104,105]

Three-dimensional time-of-flight camera measures depth movement with the camera to derive a respiratory effort signal to monitor respiration. An initial study demonstrated strong correlation (r 0.88; $P = .0001$) with RIP event detection, but it was not validated for central events.[106,107]

At this time, the standard of care for CSA detection irrespective of the underlying etiology is dual RIP belts. Some of the newer modalities may serve a role in screening or flagging potential underlying central events but not for definitive diagnosis.

CENTRAL SLEEP APNEA EPIDEMIOLOGY

CSA is relatively rare occurring in less than 1% of the general population,[14,108] but higher prevalences are reported (5.5%) in a sleep clinic population.[109] The failure of many sleep laboratories to score the central hypopneas likely impacts the reported prevalence rates. A 4-fold higher rates of CSA was reported when there was systematic central hypopnea scoring (19.7 vs 4.6%).[14] Higher prevalence rates of CSA occur in patients with comorbid HF with and without preserved ejection fraction (13%–44%),[110,111] atrial fibrillation (10%),[112] renal failure (15%),[113] stroke (8%–12%),[114] or chronic opioid use (24%).[115] CSA has a male predominance and rises in prevalence above the age of 60 to 65 years.[116–118] Race-stratified CSA data are absent, but indirect data from the MESA cohort suggest that older black males may be more at risk of CSA.[119]

CENTRAL SLEEP APNEA CLASSIFICATION, DIAGNOSIS, AND CLINICAL FEATURES

A CSA disorder is deemed to be present if the AHI is greater than 5 events per hour during sleep and greater than 50% of the events are central in nature. The arbitrary cut-offs used for defining mild (5 to <15 events/h), moderate (≤15 to <30 events/h), and severe (≥30) CSA in adults mirror those for OSA but are not based on the evidence of clinical significance.[120] In children, the cut-off values for the presence of CSA and severity differ (see Indra Narang and colleagues' article, "Central Sleep apnea and hypoventilation in children," in this issue). The International Classification of Sleep Disorders (ICSD-3-TR) further classifies CSA based on the presence of underlying comorbidities.[121] Although, an alternative approach classifies CSA based on the presence or absence of hypercapnia (partial pressure of carbon dioxide [P_{CO_2}] ≥ 45 mm Hg).[122] Lastly, Javaheri and colleagues proposed a pathophysiological classification, whereby the CSA subtypes are classified based on high LG (a measure of ventilatory stability) or dysfunction of respiratory rhythm generation[47] (**Table 3**).

A CSA disorder is associated with the presence of sleepiness, difficulty with sleep initiation or maintenance, frequent awakenings or nonrestorative sleep, awakening with shortness of breath, or witnessed apneas.[121] There may also be symptoms attributable to the underlying etiology or sequelae of hypercapnia such as muscle weakness, dyspnea, morning headaches, or peripheral edema and signs of pulmonary hypertension.

When evaluating CSA determination of the underlying etiology can guide management strategies, as these are often directed at the underlying cause (**Fig. 5**). The clinical approach can start with the assessment of blood gas tensions to stratify patients into those with or without hypercapnia and the subgroups of "can't breathe, won't breathe, and shouldn't breathe."[122] This equates to defects with the respiratory neuromuscular apparatus, the respiratory control system, and instability and fluctuations of an intact respiratory control system, respectively. However, avoidance of an assessment of CO2 may be feasible in some patients if one starts first with assessing the context in which the CSA occurs, for example, high altitude, during the treatment of OSA with positive airway pressure. Second, the pattern of CSA on the PSG may be informative (**Fig. 6**). A crescendo-decrescendo pattern (CSR) on the RIP with varying cycle length is often indicative of HF with longer cycle lengths in those with more severe HF. However, it is not pathognomonic, and a CSR pattern is also associated with atrial fibrillation, stroke, or brainstem pathology. This compares to short

Table 3
Classification of CSA subtypes in adults and children

ICSD-3-TR Classification	Alternative Clinical Classification	Pathophysiological Classification
CSA AHI $\geq$ 5, >50% central events	CSA AHI $\geq$ 5, >50% central events	CSA AHI $\geq$ 5, >50% central events
CSA due to a medical disorder *(without CSB)*	*Hypercapnic ($Pco_2 \geq 45$)*	*High loop gain/increased controller gain*
CSA due to high-altitude periodic breathing	*Primary* Central alveolar hypoventilation syndrome	Heart failure Atrial fibrillation
CSA with Cheyne-Stokes Breathing (CSB) *Presence of atrial fibrillation/heart failure or a neurologic disorder*	*Secondary* Cerebrovascular disease	High altitude Idiopathic
CSA due to a medication or substance	Neuromuscular disease	Acromegaly
Primary CSA	Developmental or degenerative disease	Treatment emergent
Primary CSA of prematurity	Brainstem tumors	Chronic renal failure
Primary CSA of infancy	Hypothyroid	Drugs
Treatment-emergent CSA	Obesity hypoventilation syndrome	
	Nonhypercapnic/normocapnic ($Pco_2 < 45$) *Primary* Idiopathic CSA *Secondary* *CSA with CSR due to heart failure* *Atrial fibrillation* *Treatment emergent CSA* *Renal failure* *High altitude* *Respiratory depressants* *Cerebrovascular disease* *Acromegaly*	*High loop gain/increased plant gain* Chronic hypercapnia Alveolar hypoventilation Congenital and primary Brainstem and spinal cord disorders Neuromuscular disorder Spinal cord disorders *Failure of rhythm generation* Drugs Neurodegenerative disorders Brainstem disorders Bilateral diaphragmatic paralysis

Abbreviations: CSA, central sleep apnea; CSB, Cheyne-Stokes breathing; CSR, Cheyne-Stokes respiration; Pco_2, partial pressure of carbon dioxide.

central events with a regular pattern in those with idiopathic CSA or an irregular pattern in patients on respiratory depressants (eg, opioids). High-altitude CSA also has a CSR pattern with a short cycle length. This highlights the importance of context in conjunction with the relevant clinical information. If the context, pattern, and available clinical information are not informative then one should proceed to evaluate for the presence or absence of hypercapnia. For those with hypercapnia, the potential etiologies include neurodegenerative or neurologic disease, chest wall disease, or respiratory depressant medications. In the absence of identifiable causes, the potential causes include primary central alveolar hypoventilation or more frequently obesity hypoventilation syndrome. For those with nonhypercapnic CSA, if there is no systemic disease (renal disease, endocrine, and cardiac disease) then the etiology is idiopathic CSA. The investigations to be considered include renal function, thyroid function, NT-proBNP, cardiac echocardiogram, electrocardiogram, neuroimaging (MRI brain), pulmonary function testing including assessment of muscle function (maximal inspiratory and expiratory pressures, peak cough flow, vital capacity erect, and supine), electromyography, and nerve conduction studies.

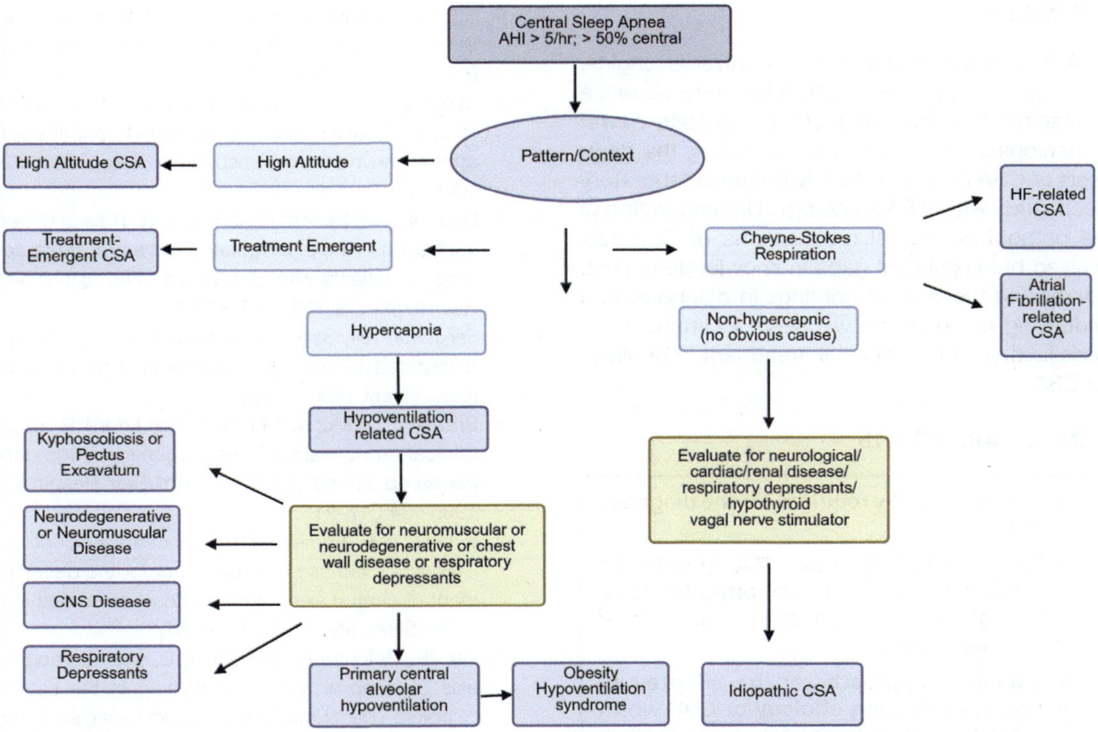

Fig. 5. Algorithm demonstrating a diagnostic approach to central sleep apnea. CSA, central sleep apnea; hypercapnia, arterial partial pressure of carbon dioxide $\geq$ 45 mm Hg. (Created in BioRender. Ryan, C. (2026) https://BioRender.com/mhmznew.)

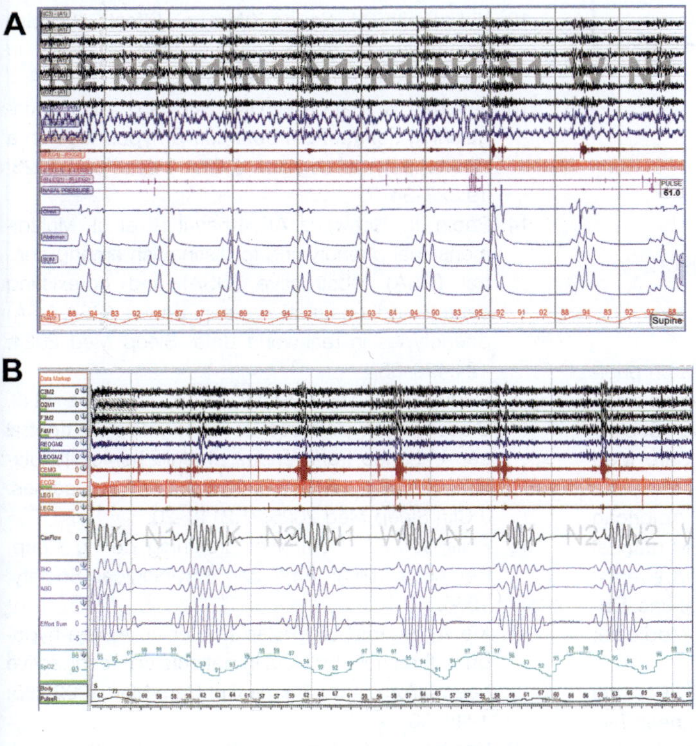

Fig. 6. (*A*) Polysomnographic tracing of central apneas during stage N1/N2 sleep from a patient with opioid-induced central sleep apnea. There is no airflow as illustrated by the nasal pressure transducer recording and an absence of rib cage (chest RIP) and abdominal (abdominal RIP) motion. Note the typical short apnea-hyperpnea cycle duration (ie, 30–35 seconds) with cyclical mild oxygen desaturations that contrasts with the long cycle duration in CSR-CSA shown. (*B*) Polysomnographic tracing of Cheyne-Stokes respiration with central sleep apnea pattern (CSR-CSA) during stage N2 sleep. There is an absence of rib cage (chest RIP) and abdominal (abdominal RIP) motion as illustrated by the chest, abdominal, and SUM respitrace recordings. There is no airflow as illustrated by the nasal pressure transducer recording. Note the typical long apnea-hyperpnea cycle duration with prolonged crescendo-decrescendo pattern of hyperpnea. Apneas are accompanied by cyclical mild oxygen desaturations. EEG electrocardiogram, electroencephalogram; EMG, electromyogram; EOG, electrooculogram; RIP, respitrace; SpO2, pulse oxygen saturation. *5-minute recording*.

SUMMARY

CSA is a complex disorder with diverse origins, characterized by a recurrent temporary absence of respiratory effort during sleep. Despite newer technologies for the diagnosis of SBDs, the diagnosis of CSA continues to rely on the in-laboratory sleep study with RIP technology. Understanding of the pathophysiological mechanisms of CSA has evolved but significant gaps in knowledge persist. Addressing these short comings in diagnosis and underlying mechanisms will serve to improve the classification and potential treatment modalities for CSA.

CLINICS CARE POINTS

- Full PSG is currently required for the diagnosis of CSA.
- Although relatively rare CSA should be considered in those with comorbid HF, renal failure, atrial fibrillation, at high altitude or chronic opioid users.
- A pragmatic approach can be adopted to assess the underlying etiology of CSA, which includes evaluation of the context (e.g. medications, comorbid conditions), pattern and if necessary blood gas tensions.
- Treatment modalities are determined by the underlying etiology of CSA.

FUNDING

No funding.

DISCLOSURE

No conflict of interest related to this project.

REFERENCES

1. Orr JE, Ayappa I, Eckert DJ, et al. Research priorities for patients with heart failure and central sleep apnea. An official American thoracic Society research statement. Am J Respir Crit Care Med 2021;203:e11–24.
2. Troester MMQS, Berry et al; for the American Academy of Sleep Medicine. The AASM manual for the socring of sleep and associated events: rule, terminology and technical specifications. Darien (IL): American Academy of Sleep Medicine; 2023.
3. Pinna GD, Dacosto E, Maestri R, et al. Postural changes in lung volumes in patients with heart failure and Cheyne-Stokes respiration: relationship with sleep apnea severity. Sleep Med 2023;101:154–61.
4. Sahlin C, Svanborg E, Stenlund H, et al. Cheyne-Stokes respiration and supine dependency. Eur Respir J 2005;25:829–33.
5. Szollosi I, Roebuck T, Thompson B, et al. Lateral sleeping position reduces severity of central sleep apnea/Cheyne-Stokes respiration. Sleep 2006;29:1045–51.
6. Naughton M, Benard D, Tam A, et al. Role of hyperventilation in the pathogenesis of central sleep apneas in patients with congestive heart failure. Am Rev Respir Dis 1993;148:330–8.
7. Ferguson KA, Strong MJ, Ahmad D, et al. Sleep-disordered breathing in amyotrophic lateral sclerosis. Chest 1996;110:664–9.
8. Bradley TD, McNicholas WT, Rutherford R, et al. Clinical and physiologic heterogeneity of the central sleep apnea syndrome. Am Rev Respir Dis 1986;134:217–21.
9. Walker JM, Farney RJ, Rhondeau SM, et al. Chronic opioid use is a risk factor for the development of central sleep apnea and ataxic breathing. J Clin Sleep Med 2007;3:455–61.
10. Orr JE, Malhotra A, Gruenberg E, et al. Pathogenesis of sleep-disordered breathing in the setting of opioid use: a multiple mediation analysis using physiology. Sleep 2024;47.
11. Hanly PJ, Millar TW, Steljes DG, et al. Respiration and abnormal sleep in patients with congestive heart failure. Chest 1989;96:480–8.
12. Xi L, Smith CA, Saupe KW, et al. Effects of rapid-eye-movement sleep on the apneic threshold in dogs. J Appl Physiol 1993;75:1129–39.
13. Javaheri S, Rapoport DM, Schwartz AR. Distinguishing central from obstructive hypopneas on a clinical polysomnogram. J Clin Sleep Med 2023;19:823–34.
14. Pepin JL, Schwartz AR, Khayat R, et al. Multidimensional phenotyping to distinguish among central (CSA), obstructive (OSA) and co-existing central and obstructive sleep apnea (CSA-OSA) phenotypes in real-world data. Sleep Med 2024;124:426–33.
15. Dupuy-McCauley K, Schwartz AR, Javaheri S, et al. Classifying hypopneas as obstructive or central can enhance transvenous phrenic nerve stimulation therapy patient selection and outcomes. J Clin Sleep Med 2025;21:2113–20.
16. Phillipson EA. Control of breathing during sleep. Bethesda (MD): American Phyiological Society; 1986.
17. Xie A, Skatrud JB, Puleo DS, et al. Apnea-hypopnea threshold for CO2 in patients with congestive heart failure. Am J Respir Crit Care Med 2002;165:1245–50.
18. Dempsey JA. Crossing the apnoeic threshold: causes and consequences. Exp Physiol 2005;90:13–24.

19. Skatrud JB, Dempsey JA. Interaction of sleep state and chemical stimuli in sustaining rhythmic ventilation. J Appl Physiol 1983;55:813–22.
20. Dempsey JA, Smith CA, Przybylowski T, et al. The ventilatory responsiveness to CO(2) below eupnoea as a determinant of ventilatory stability in sleep. J Physiol 2004;560:1–11.
21. Xie A, Wong B, Phillipson EA, et al. Interaction of hyperventilation and arousal in the pathogenesis of idiopathic central sleep apnea. Am J Respir Crit Care Med 1994;150:489–95.
22. Xie A, Rutherford R, Rankin F, et al. Hypocapnia and increased ventilatory responsiveness in patients with idiopathic central sleep apnea. Am J Respir Crit Care Med 1995;152:1950–5.
23. Xie A, Rankin F, Rutherford R, et al. Effects of inhaled CO2 and added dead space on idiopathic central sleep apnea. J Appl Physiol 1997;82:918–26.
24. Lorenzi-Filho G, Rankin F, Bies I, et al. Effects of inhaled carbon dioxide and oxygen on cheyne-stokes respiration in patients with heart failure. Am J Respir Crit Care Med 1999;159:1490–8.
25. Khoo MC. Determinants of ventilatory instability and variability. Respir Physiol 2000;122:167–82.
26. Cherniack NS, Longobardo GS. Mathematical models of periodic breathing and their usefulness in understanding cardiovascular and respiratory disorders. Exp Physiol 2006;91:295–305.
27. Solin P, Roebuck T, Johns DP, et al. Peripheral and central ventilatory responses in central sleep apnea with and without congestive heart failure. Am J Respir Crit Care Med 2000;162:2194–200.
28. Sands SA, Mebrate Y, Edwards BA, et al. Resonance as the mechanism of daytime periodic breathing in patients with heart failure. Am J Respir Crit Care Med 2017;195:237–46.
29. Javaheri S, McKane SW, Cameron N, et al. In patients with heart failure the burden of central sleep apnea increases in the late sleep hours. Sleep 2019;42.
30. Giannoni A, Gentile F, Navari A, et al. Contribution of the lung to the genesis of cheyne-stokes respiration in heart failure: plant gain beyond chemoreflex gain and circulation time. J Am Heart Assoc 2019;8:e012419.
31. Miyamoto T, Inagaki M, Takaki H, et al. Integrated characterization of the human chemoreflex system controlling ventilation, using an equilibrium diagram. Eur J Appl Physiol 2004;93:340–6.
32. Chowdhuri S, Pranathiageswaran S, Loomis-King H, et al. Aging is associated with increased propensity for central apnea during NREM sleep. J Appl Physiol 2018;124:83–90.
33. Zhou XS, Shahabuddin S, Zahn BR, et al. Effect of gender on the development of hypocapnic apnea/hypopnea during NREM sleep. J Appl Physiol 2000;89:192–9.
34. Pinna GD, Robbi E, Terzaghi M, et al. Temporal relationship between arousals and Cheyne-Stokes respiration with central sleep apnea in heart failure patients. Clin Neurophysiol 2018;129:1955–63.
35. Pinna GD, Robbi E, Bruschi C, et al. Interaction between arousals and ventilation during cheyne-stokes respiration in heart failure patients: insights from breath-by-breath analysis. Front Med 2021;8:742458.
36. Guilleminault C, Quera-Salva MA, Nino-Murcia G, et al. Central sleep apnea and partial obstruction of the upper airway. Ann Neurol 1987;21:465–9.
37. Badr MS, Toiber F, Skatrud JB, et al. Pharyngeal narrowing/occlusion during central sleep apnea. J Appl Physiol 1995;78:1806–15.
38. Kasai T, Motwani SS, Yumino D, et al. Contrasting effects of lower body positive pressure on upper airways resistance and partial pressure of carbon dioxide in men with heart failure and obstructive or central sleep apnea. J Am Coll Cardiol 2013;61:1157–66.
39. Bhakta NR, McGowan A, Ramsey KA, et al. European Respiratory Society/American Thoracic Society technical statement: standardisation of the measurement of lung volumes, 2023 update. Eur Respir J 2023;62:2201519.
40. Francis DP, Willson K, Davies LC, et al. Quantitative general theory for periodic breathing in chronic heart failure and its clinical implications. Circulation 2000;102:2214–21.
41. Malte CL, Malte H, Wang T. Periodic ventilation: consequences for the bodily CO2 stores and gas exchange efficiency. Respir Physiol Neurobiol 2016;231:63–74.
42. Yumino D, Redolfi S, Ruttanaumpawan P, et al. Nocturnal rostral fluid shift: a unifying concept for the pathogenesis of obstructive and central sleep apnea in men with heart failure. Circulation 2010;121:1598–605.
43. White LH, Bradley TD. Role of nocturnal rostral fluid shift in the pathogenesis of obstructive and central sleep apnoea. J Physiol 2013;591:1179–93.
44. Thompson WO, Thompson PK, Dailey ME. The effect of posture upon the composition and volume of the blood in man. Proc Natl Acad Sci U S A 1928;14:94–8.
45. Lyons OD, Inami T, Perger E, et al. The effect of fluid overload on sleep apnoea severity in haemodialysis patients. Eur Respir J 2017;49.
46. Lyons OD, Chan CT, Yadollahi A, et al. Effect of ultrafiltration on sleep apnea and sleep structure in patients with end-stage renal disease. Am J Respir Crit Care Med 2015;191:1287–94.
47. Javaheri S, Badr MS. Central sleep apnea: pathophysiologic classification. Sleep 2023;46.
48. Bascom AT, Sankari A, Badr MS. Spinal cord injury is associated with enhanced peripheral chemoreflex sensitivity. Physiological reports 2016;4.

49. Sankari A, Bascom AT, Chowdhuri S, et al. Tetraplegia is a risk factor for central sleep apnea. J Appl Physiol 2014;116:345–53.
50. Ponikowski P, Anker SD, Chua TP, et al. Oscillatory breathing patterns during wakefulness in patients with chronic heart failure: clinical implications and role of augmented peripheral chemosensitivity. Circulation 1999;100:2418–24.
51. Sun SY, Wang W, Zucker IH, et al. Enhanced peripheral chemoreflex function in conscious rabbits with pacing-induced heart failure. J Appl Physiol 1999;86:1264–72.
52. Conde SV, Monteiro EC, Sacramento JF. Purines and carotid body: new roles in pathological conditions. Front Pharmacol 2017;8:913.
53. Marcus NJ, Del Rio R, Ding Y, et al. KLF2 mediates enhanced chemoreflex sensitivity, disordered breathing and autonomic dysregulation in heart failure. J Physiol 2018;596:3171–85.
54. Solin P, Bergin P, Richardson M, et al. Influence of pulmonary capillary wedge pressure on central apnea in heart failure. Circulation 1999; 99:1574–9.
55. Georgiadis D, Sievert M, Cencetti S, et al. Cerebrovascular reactivity is impaired in patients with cardiac failure. Eur Heart J 2000;21:407–13.
56. Xie A, Skatrud JB, Khayat R, et al. Cerebrovascular response to carbon dioxide in patients with congestive heart failure. Am J Respir Crit Care Med 2005; 172:371–8.
57. Hall MJ, Xie A, Rutherford R, et al. Cycle length of periodic breathing in patients with and without heart failure. Am J Respir Crit Care Med 1996; 154:376–81.
58. Feldman JL, Del Negro CA. Looking for inspiration: new perspectives on respiratory rhythm. Nat Rev Neurosci 2006;7:232–42.
59. McKay LC, Feldman JL. Unilateral ablation of prebotzinger complex disrupts breathing during sleep but not wakefulness. Am J Respir Crit Care Med 2008;178:89–95.
60. Orem J. The nature of the wakefulness stimulus for breathing. Prog Clin Biol Res 1990;345:23–30 [discussion: 31].
61. Phillipson EABG. Control of breathing during sleep. In: Cherniack NSWJ, editor. Handbook of physiology. Bethesda (MD): American Physiological Society; 1986. p. 649–89.
62. Lin M, Krishnan AV, Eckert DJ. Central sleep apnea in multiple sclerosis: a pilot study. Sleep & breathing = Schlaf & Atmung 2017;21:691–6.
63. Ferre A, Poca MA, de la Calzada MD, et al. Sleep-related breathing disorders in Chiari malformation type 1: a prospective study of 90 patients. Sleep 2017;40.
64. Bourke SC, Gibson GJ. Sleep and breathing in neuromuscular disease. Eur Respir J 2002;19:1194–201.
65. Javaheri S, Randerath WJ, Safwan Badr M, et al. Medication-induced central sleep apnea: a unifying concept. Sleep 2024;47.
66. Baertsch NA, Bush NE, Burgraff NJ, et al. Dual mechanisms of opioid-induced respiratory depression in the inspiratory rhythm-generating network. eLife 2021;10.
67. Varga AG, Reid BT, Kieffer BL, et al. Differential impact of two critical respiratory centres in opioid-induced respiratory depression in awake mice. J Physiol 2020;598:189–205.
68. Saunders SE, Baekey DM, Levitt ES. Fentanyl effects on respiratory neuron activity in the dorsolateral pons. J Neurophysiol 2022;128:1117–32.
69. Teichtahl H, Wang D, Cunnington D, et al. Ventilatory responses to hypoxia and hypercapnia in stable methadone maintenance treatment patients. Chest 2005;128:1339–47.
70. Wang D, Yee BJ, Grunstein RR, et al. Chronic opioid use and central sleep apnea, where are we now and where to go? A state of the art review. Anesth Analg 2021;132:1244–53.
71. Practice parameters for the use of portable recording in the assessment of obstructive sleep apnea. Standards of practice committee of the American Sleep Disorders Association. Sleep 1994;17:372–7.
72. Flemons WW, Littner MR, Rowley JA, et al. Home diagnosis of sleep apnea: a systematic review of the literature. An evidence review cosponsored by the American Academy of Sleep Medicine, the American College of Chest Physicians, and the American Thoracic Society. Chest 2003;124:1543–79.
73. Riha RL, Celmina M, Cooper B, et al. ERS technical standards for using type III devices (limited channel studies) in the diagnosis of sleep disordered breathing in adults and children. Eur Respir J 2023;61.
74. Serrano Alarcon A, Martinez Madrid N, Seepold R. A minimum set of physiological parameters to diagnose obstructive sleep apnea syndrome using non-invasive portable monitors. A Systematic Review Life (Basel) 2021;11.
75. Collop NA, Anderson WM, Boehlecke B, et al. Portable monitoring task force of the American Academy of Sleep M. Clinical guidelines for the use of unattended portable monitors in the diagnosis of obstructive sleep apnea in adult patients. Portable Monitoring Task Force of the American Academy of Sleep Medicine. J Clin Sleep Med 2007;3:737–47.
76. Weinreich G, Armitstead J, Topfer V, et al. Validation of ApneaLink as screening device for Cheyne-Stokes respiration. Sleep 2009;32:553–7.
77. Quintana-Gallego E, Villa-Gil M, Carmona-Bernal C, et al. Home respiratory polygraphy for diagnosis

of sleep-disordered breathing in heart failure. Eur Respir J 2004;24:443–8.
78. Pinna GD, Robbi E, Pizza F, et al. Can cardiorespiratory polygraphy replace portable polysomnography in the assessment of sleep-disordered breathing in heart failure patients? Sleep & breathing = Schlaf & Atmung 2014;18:475–82.
79. Tung PH, Hsieh MJ, Chuang LP, et al. Efficacy of portable sleep monitoring device in diagnosing central sleep apnea in patients with congestive heart failure. Front Neurol 2022;13:1043413.
80. Badr MS, Khayat RN, Allam JS, et al. Treatment of central sleep apnea in adults: an American Academy of Sleep Medicine clinical practice guideline. J Clin Sleep Med 2025;21:2181–91.
81. Kushida CA, Giacomini A, Lee MK, et al. Technical protocol for the use of esophageal manometry in the diagnosis of sleep-related breathing disorders. Sleep Med 2002;3:163–73.
82. Cantineau JP, Escourrou P, Sartene R, et al. Accuracy of respiratory inductive plethysmography during wakefulness and sleep in patients with obstructive sleep apnea. Chest 1992;102:1145–51.
83. Sackner MA, Watson H, Belsito AS, et al. Calibration of respiratory inductive plethysmograph during natural breathing. J Appl Physiol 1989;66:410–20.
84. Banzett RB, Mahan ST, Garner DM, et al. A simple and reliable method to calibrate respiratory magnetometers and respitrace. J Appl Physiol 1995;79:2169–76.
85. Montazeri K, Jonsson SA, Agustsson JS, et al. The design of RIP belts impacts the reliability and quality of the measured respiratory signals. Sleep & breathing = Schlaf & Atmung 2021;25:1535–41.
86. VVTea. A portable respiratory monitor using respiratory inductive plethysmography, 4th international conference on biomedical engineering in Vietnam, IFMBE proceedings. Vietnam: Springer Nature; 2013. p. 222–5.
87. Finnsson E, Arnardottir E, Montazeri K, et al. Respiratory inductance plethysmography to quantify changes in ventilation in obstructive sleep apnea. IEEE Trans Biomed Eng 2026;73:1943–52.
88. Finnsson E, Erlingsson E, Hlynsson HD, et al. Detecting arousals and sleep from respiratory inductance plethysmography. Sleep & breathing = Schlaf & Atmung 2025;29:155.
89. Rahman MS, Chowdhury S, Rasheduzzaman M, et al. Artificial intelligence-based algorithms and healthcare applications of respiratory inductance plethysmography: a systematic review. Algorithms 2024;17:1–32.
90. Vaughn CM, Clemmons P. Piezoelectric belts as a method for measuring chest and abdominal movement for obstructive sleep apnea diagnosis. Neurodiagn J 2012;52:275–80.
91. Koo BB, Drummond C, Surovec S, et al. Validation of a polyvinylidene fluoride impedance sensor for respiratory event classification during polysomnography. J Clin Sleep Med 2011;7:479–85.
92. Griffiths AG, Patwari PP, Loghmanee DA, et al. Validation of polyvinylidene fluoride impedance sensor for respiratory event classification during polysomnography in children. J Clin Sleep Med 2017;13:259–65.
93. Vulcan RS, Andre S, Bruyneel M. Photoplethysmography in normal and pathological sleep. Sensors (Basel) 2021;21.
94. Lazazzera R, Deviaene M, Varon C, et al. Detection and classification of sleep apnea and hypopnea using PPG and SpO (2) signals. IEEE Trans Biomed Eng 2021;68:1496–506.
95. Massie F, Vits S, Khachatryan A, et al. Central sleep apnea detection by means of finger photoplethysmography. IEEE J Transl Eng Health Med 2023;11:126–36.
96. Pillar G, Berall M, Berry R, et al. Detecting central sleep apnea in adult patients using WatchPAT-a multicenter validation study. Sleep & breathing = Schlaf & Atmung 2020;24:387–98.
97. Amir O, Barak-Shinar D, Henry A, et al. Photoplethysmography as a single source for analysis of sleep-disordered breathing in patients with severe cardiovascular disease. J Sleep Res 2012;21:94–100.
98. Somers VK, Dyken ME, Mark AL, et al. Sympathetic-nerve activity during sleep in normal subjects. N Engl J Med 1993;328:303–7.
99. Cui J, Huang Z, Wu J, et al. Cardiopulmonary resonance function and Indices-A quantitative measurement for respiratory sinus arrhythmia. Front Physiol 2020;11:867.
100. Thomas RJ, Mietus JE, Peng CK, et al. An electrocardiogram-based technique to assess cardiopulmonary coupling during sleep. Sleep 2005;28:1151–61.
101. Al Ashry HS, Ni Y, Thomas RJ. Cardiopulmonary sleep spectrograms open a novel window into sleep biology-implications for health and disease. Front Neurosci 2021;15:755464.
102. Al Ashry HS, Hilmisson H, Ni Y, et al. Automated apnea-hypopnea index from oximetry and spectral analysis of cardiopulmonary coupling. Ann Am Thorac Soc 2021;18:876–83.
103. Thomas RJ, Mietus JE, Peng CK, et al. Differentiating obstructive from central and complex sleep apnea using an automated electrocardiogram-based method. Sleep 2007;30:1756–69.
104. Edouard P, Campo D, Bartet P, et al. Validation of the withings sleep analyzer, an under-the-mattress device for the detection of moderate-severe sleep apnea syndrome. J Clin Sleep Med 2021;17:1217–27.

105. Siyahjani F, Kalenyk K, Garcia-Molina G, et al. Validating a smart bed against polysomnography for sleep apnea detection. Sci Rep 2025;15:23607.
106. Coronel C, Wiesmeyr C, Garn H, et al. Measurement of respiratory effort in sleep by 3D camera and respiratory inductance plethysmography. Somnologie 2019;23:86–92.
107. Coronel C, Wiesmeyr C, Garn H, et al. 3D camera and pulse oximeter for respiratory events detection. IEEE J Biomed Health Inform 2021;25:181–8.
108. Donovan LM, Kapur VK. Prevalence and characteristics of central compared to obstructive sleep apnea: analyses from the sleep heart health study cohort. Sleep (New York, NY) 2016;39:1353–9.
109. Patel SR, Genuardi MV, DeSensi R, et al. Real world characteristics of central sleep apnea: a review of 29,000 consecutive patients undergoing polysomnography. Sleep & breathing = Schlaf & Atmung 2025;29:296.
110. Wang T, Yu FC, Wei Q, et al. Prevalence and clinical characteristics of sleep-disordered breathing in patients with heart failure of different left ventricular ejection fractions. Sleep & breathing = Schlaf & Atmung 2023;27:245–53.
111. Javaheri S, Barbe F, Campos-Rodriguez F, et al. Sleep apnea: types, mechanisms, and clinical cardiovascular consequences. J Am Coll Cardiol 2017;69:841–58.
112. Kadhim K, Middeldorp ME, Elliott AD, et al. Prevalence and assessment of sleep-disordered breathing in patients with atrial fibrillation: a systematic review and meta-analysis. Can J Cardiol 2021;37: 1846–56.
113. Strotmann J, Fox H, Bitter T, et al. Characteristics of sleep-disordered breathing in patients with atrial fibrillation and preserved left ventricular ejection fraction. Clin Res Cardiol 2018;107:120–9.
114. Baillieul S, Dekkers M, Brill AK, et al. Sleep apnoea and ischaemic stroke: current knowledge and future directions. Lancet Neurol 2022;21:78–88.
115. Mubashir T, Nagappa M, Esfahanian N, et al. Prevalence of sleep-disordered breathing in opioid users with chronic pain: a systematic review and meta-analysis. J Clin Sleep Med 2020;16:961–9.
116. Bixler EO, Vgontzas AN, Ten Have T, et al. Effects of age on sleep apnea in men: I. Prevalence and severity. Am J Respir Crit Care Med 1998;157: 144–8.
117. Johansson P, Alehagen U, Svanborg E, et al. Sleep disordered breathing in an elderly community-living population: relationship to cardiac function, insomnia symptoms and daytime sleepiness. Sleep Med 2009;10:1005–11.
118. Young T, Shahar E, Nieto FJ, et al, Sleep Heart Health Study Research G. Predictors of sleep-disordered breathing in community-dwelling adults: the sleep heart health study. Arch Intern Med 2002;162: 893–900.
119. Sands SA, Alex RM, Mann D, et al. Pathophysiology underlying demographic and obesity determinants of sleep apnea severity. Ann Am Thorac Soc 2023;20:440–9.
120. Fleetham J, Ayas N, Bradley D, et al. Canadian thoracic society guidelines: diagnosis and treatment of sleep disordered breathing in adults. Cancer Res J 2006;13:387–92.
121. Medicine AAoS. International classification of sleep disorders. Darien (IL): American Academy of Sleep Medicine; 2023.
122. Ryan C, Bradley TD. Central sleep apnea. In: Broaddus VC, editor. Textbook of respiratory medicine. Canada: Elsevier; 2022. p. 1670–86.
123. Horner RLM, A. Control of Breathing and Upper Airways During Sleep. In: V. Courtney Broaddus MD (Author) JDEME, Talmadge E. King Jr MD (Editor), Stephen C. Lazarus MD (Editor), Kathleen F. Sarmiento MD (Editor), Lynn M. Schnapp MD (Editor), Renee D. Stapleton MD PhD (Editor), Michael B. Gotway MD (Editor) editor. Murray and Nadel's Textbook of Respiratory Medicine, 7th ed. Canada: Elselvier; 2016. p. 1511–1526.

Central Sleep Apnea in Cardiovascular Diseases

Sayaki Ishiwata, MD, PhD[a], T. Douglas Bradley, MD[a,b,c,*]

KEYWORDS

- Central sleep apnea (CSA) • Cardiovascular diseases (CVDs) • Heart failure (HF)
- Atrial fibrillation (AF) • Cerebrovascular accidents (CVA) • Apnea threshold
- Sleep-related breathing • Pathophysiology

KEY POINTS

- Central sleep apnea (CSA) is most commonly associated with cardiovascular diseases, particularly heart failure, atrial fibrillation, and cerebrovascular accidents.
- Central apneas generally occur during sleep when arterial CO_2 levels ($Paco_2$) fall below the apnea threshold due to various stimuli, despite variations in underlying pathophysiology.
- In patients with CSA linked to cardiovascular conditions, $Paco_2$ levels are typically normal or low. This article focuses on epidemiology, clinical manifestations, prognosis and treatment.

INTRODUCTION

Central sleep apnea (CSA) most commonly occurs in association with cardiovascular diseases (CVDs), and in particular heart failure (HF), atrial fibrillation (AF) and cerebrovascular accidents (CVAs). A detailed discussion of the pathophysiology of CSA in the setting of CVD is provided in another article (see Clodagh M. Ryan and T. Douglas Bradley's article, "Central Sleep Apnea: Pathophysiology, Classification and Diagnosis," in this issue) and will not be covered in any detail herein. Although its pathophysiology varies, in general, central apneas occur when the partial pressure of arterial CO_2 ($Paco_2$) falls below the apnea threshold during sleep due to various stimuli.[1,2] In patients with CSA in the setting of HF, AF and CVA are generally either normo-capneic or hypocapneic, but not hypercapneic.[3] In this article, we will focus on the epidemiology, clinical manifestations, prognostic implications, and treatment of CSA in the setting of CVD.

CENTRAL SLEEP APNEA IN HEART FAILURE

Epidemiology

Sleep-disordered breathing (SDB) is highly prevalent in patients with HF, with both obstructive sleep apnea (OSA) and CSA frequently observed across the spectrum of HF phenotypes. Contemporary studies suggest that approximately 50% to 70% of patients with chronic HF exhibit some form of SDB, although prevalence estimates vary according to patient selection, diagnostic methodology, and definitions used for respiratory events. Among patients with HF with reduced ejection fraction (HFrEF), CSA accompanied by Cheyne–Stokes respiration (CSA-CSR) is common, occurring in approximately 20% to 40% of patients. However, OSA appears to be more prevalent than CSA in this population.[4–6] To complicate matters, CSA-CSR and OSA often co-exist in patients with HFrEF, although one type generally predominates.[6] In addition, the predominant type of SDB can shift over time: those with predominantly OSA may

[a] Sleep Research Laboratories of the University Health Network, Toronto Rehabilitation Institute (KITE), Toronto General Hospital, University of Toronto, Toronto, Ontario, Canada; [b] Department of Medicine, University Health Network, Sinai Health, University of Toronto, Toronto, Ontario, Canada; [c] Toronto General Hospital Research Institute, Toronto, Ontario, Canada
* Corresponding author. University Health Network Toronto General Hospital, 200 Elizabeth Street, Room 9N-943, Toronto, ON M5R3P7, Canada.
E-mail address: Douglas.Bradley@utoronto.ca

Sleep Med Clin 21 (2026) 317–331
https://doi.org/10.1016/j.jsmc.2026.06.005
1556-407X/26/

Abbreviations	
AASM	American Academy of Sleep Medicine
ADVENT-HF	Adaptive Servo-ventilation for Sleep-disordered Breathing in Patients with Heart Failure with Reduced Ejection Fraction
AF	atrial fibrillation
AHI	apnea-hypopnea index
ASV	adaptive servo-ventilation
CANPAP	Canadian Continuous Positive Airway Pressure for Patients with Central Sleep Apnea and Heart Failure
CPAP	continuous positive airway pressure
CSA	central sleep apnea
CSR	Cheyne–Stokes respiration
CVA	cerebrovascular accident
CVD	cardiovascular disease
EEG	Electroencephalogram
EMG_{sm}	submental electromyogram
EMG_{at}	anterior tibialis electromyogram
EKG	Electrocardiogram
ESS	Epworth Sleepiness Scale
HF	heart failure
HFpEF	heart failure and preserved ejection fraction
HFrEF	heart failure with reduced ejection fraction
HR	hazard ratio
ICSA	idiopathic CSA
LVEF	left ventricular ejection fraction
MLHFQ	Minnesota Living with Heart Failure Questionnaire
MV	minute ventilation
NYHA	New York Heart Association
OSA	obstructive sleep apnea
$PaCO_2$	partial pressure of arterial CO_2
PF	peak airflow
PLM	periodic leg movements
REM	rapid eye movement
SaO_2	arterial oxyhemoglobin saturation
SDB	sleep-disordered breathing

convert to predominantly to CSA-CSR if cardiac function deteriorates, and vice versa.[7,8] Nevertheless, compared to those with OSA or no SDB, those with CSA-CSR have signs of more advanced HF including older age, more male predominance, lower body mass index, lower left ventricular ejection fraction (LVEF), worse mitral regurgitation, longer circulation time, higher cardiac filling pressures, lower $Paco_2$, higher prevalence of AF, and rates of pacemaker and cardioverter-defibrillator implantation as well as higher mortality risk.[4,5,9] CSA-CSR has also been associated with adverse nonfatal clinical outcomes and may serve as a marker of disease progression in patients with chronic HF and could identify individuals who may benefit from earlier referral for advanced therapies, mechanical circulatory support, or transplantation.[9]

Compared to HFrEF, fewer studies have examined the prevalence and clinical implications of SDB in patients with HF and preserved ejection fraction (HFpEF). Similar to HFrEF, recent observational studies suggest that SDB in HFpEF is highly prevalent, often with co-existence of OSA and CSA but with one type usually predominating.[10] Whether CSA is generally associated with CSR has also not been addressed. In HFpEF, OSA appears more prevalent than CSA overall.[10–12] However, whether the predominant type of SDB can shift over time in patients with HFpEF has not been studied. As in HFrEF, this suggests some common underlying pathophysiological factors in OSA and CSA in such patients.

Data specifically addressing CSA in patients with HFpEF remain limited compared with those available for HFrEF.[13] Although SDB is common in HFpEF, most studies have focused on OSA or combined SDB populations, making the true prevalence of CSA difficult to establish. In a prospective cohort of 233 patients with HFpEF, moderate-to-severe SDB was identified in 41% of patients, with predominantly CSA observed in 14% and predominantly OSA in 27%.[14] Similarly, analyses across the spectrum of HF have demonstrated that the prevalence of central events decreases as LVEF increases, whereas obstructive events become more common. In a cohort of 700 patients with HF, nighttime central apneas were present in 66% of patients with HFrEF compared with 34% of those with HFpEF.[13] Patients with CSA in HFpEF appear more likely to exhibit markers of advanced cardiac dysfunction, including higher filling pressures, elevated natriuretic peptide concentrations, and higher rates of AF; however, the clinical phenotype and prognostic significance of CSA in HFpEF remain incompletely characterized. Further studies specifically focused on CSA are needed to define its prevalence, mechanisms, and clinical consequences in HFpEF.

Clinical Manifestations

Patients with CSA-CSR in HFrEF frequently present differently from patients with primary OSA. For example, patients with CSA often do not report snoring or excessive daytime sleepiness (EDS). Instead, patients more commonly report fragmented sleep, recurrent nocturnal awakenings, nocturnal dyspnea, and insomnia. Since they also have more advanced HF than those with OSA or no SDB, symptoms are more often attributable to the underlying HF, rather than to SDB per se, such as fatigue, impaired exercise tolerance, ankle edema, and physiologic evidence of more advanced HF. Repetitive cycles of hyperventilation and apnea may result in sleep fragmentation, reduced sleep efficiency, and impaired sleep quality.[15] Bed partners may observe periodic breathing, pauses in respiration, or restless sleep even if patients themselves remain unaware of these abnormalities.[4–6,16–18] The reason for relative absence of hypersomnolence in HFrEF-associated CSA-CSR is not well understood. However, studies in patients with HFrEF and OSA have demonstrated an inverse relationship between subjective daytime sleepiness and sympathetic nervous system activity in patients with HFrEF. This suggests that higher sympathetic activity may enhance alertness through activation of the reticular activating system and mask sleepiness due to sleep fragmentation.[19,20] Since patients with HFrEF and CSA-CSR have higher sympathetic activity than those with HFrEF but with either OSA or no SDB, the relative lack of hypersomnolence may be at least partly attributable to sympathetic activation.[19–21] Consequently, symptom severity does not necessarily correlate with the degree of nocturnal respiratory disturbance.

This "sleepiness paradox" has important clinical implications because reliance on excessive daytime sleepiness to screen for SDB may substantially underestimate clinically significant CSA-CSR in patients with HFrEF. Therefore, screening based solely on classical symptoms of OSA is insufficient in this population, and objective sleep evaluation, preferable by PSG, should be considered in patients with advanced HFrEF who have AF, recurrent HF hospitalizations, persistent fatigue and exercise limitation even in the absence of excessive daytime sleepiness.[22]

POLYSOMNOGRAPHIC AND PHYSIOLOGIC FEATURES

Polysomnographic Features of Cheyne–Stokes Respiration

Definitions and scoring of central apneas, hypopneas, and Cheyne–Stokes respiration are based on standardized American Academy of Sleep Medicine (AASM) criteria.[23] However, variability in respiratory event definitions and scoring methodology may contribute to differences in reported prevalence and phenotypic classification across studies.

The characteristic PSG pattern of CSA in HF is Cheyne–Stokes respiration, defined by cyclic crescendo–decrescendo changes in tidal volume interspersed with central apneas or hypopneas (**Fig. 1**). CSA-CSR cycle length is defined as the interval from the onset of one central apnea or hypopnea to the onset of the next event. In patients with HF, CSA-CSR cycle and hyperpnea durations are prolonged and are much longer than in those with CSA but without HF owing to longer lung-to-chemoreceptor circulation time[24–26] (see **Fig. 1**). The prolonged crescendo-decrescendo pattern of hyperpnea is related to the gradual and prolonged transmission of blood gas changes in the lungs to the peripheral and central chemoreceptors.[26]

CSR is generally considered to reflect instability in the respiratory control system and is associated with enhanced chemoreflex sensitivity, increased overnight fluid shift from the legs to the lungs with stimulation of pulmonary vagal irritant receptors and prolonged circulation time.[17,24]

CSR is primarily dependent on chemical-metabolic influences and is most prominent during non-rapid eye movement (non-REM) sleep, when ventilatory control is mainly dependent on chemical/metabolic influences. In contrast, CSA-CSR becomes less prominent in REM sleep when chemical-metabolic influences are diminished, and nonmetabolic/behavioral influences predominate. Accordingly, central apneas and hypopneas are more frequent in non-REM than in REM sleep.[1,3] In addition, overnight rostral fluid shift into the lungs during the recumbent position may contribute to hyperventilation through stimulation of pulmonary vagal irritant receptors causing hyperventilation.[27,28] Furthermore, substantial night-to-night variability in CSA-CSR severity has been demonstrated in patients with HF,[29] which emphasizes the limitation of relying on single-night polysomnography for phenotyping and severity assessment. Cyclic fluctuations in ventilation, intermittent hypoxia, arousals, and intrathoracic pressure changes may further exacerbate autonomic dysregulation and cardiovascular stress.[30]

Prognostic Implications

In patients with HFrEF, there is controversy as to whether CSA-CSR is associated with adverse cardiovascular outcomes, including increased mortality, HF hospitalization, ventricular arrhythmias, and sudden cardiac death. Some studies report such a relationship,[9,31] whereas others do not.[15,32,33] One mechanism through which CSA-CSR could contribute to adverse CV effects is sympathetic nervous system activation. HFrEF provokes sympathetic activation, and the greater this activation, the higher the mortality risk.[30] Coexisting CSA-CSR may contribute to sympathetic activation through disinhibition of sympathetic outflow by apneas and sympathetic stimulation by intermittent apnea-related hypoxia and arousals from sleep.[3] Compared to patients with HFrEF and either no SDB or OSA, those with CSA-CSR

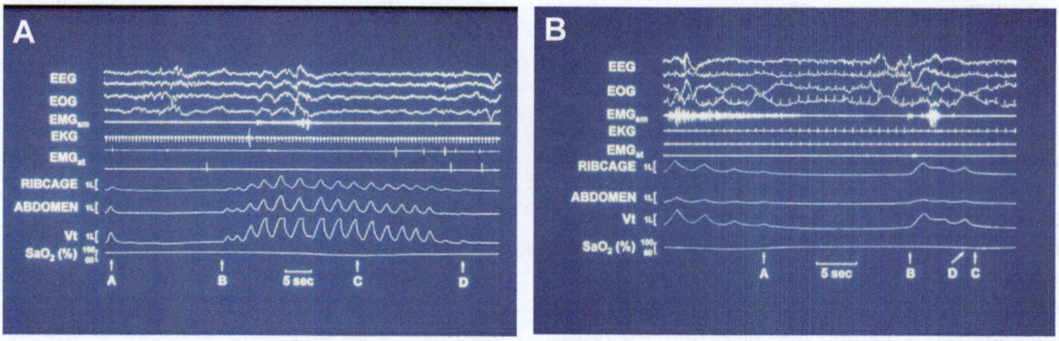

Fig. 1. (*A*) Polysomnographic recording of central sleep apnea with Cheyne–Stokes respiration (CSA-CSR) in a patient with heart failure. Note the absence of rib cage and abdominal motion when there is no tidal volume (V_t) excursion, indicating an absence of central respiratory drive. Following apnea, there is a crescendo-decrescendo pattern of V_t typical of CSA-CSR in association with a prolonged periodic cycle duration. A and B are the beginning and end of the of the apnea, respectively. C is the lowest arterial oxygen saturation (SaO_2) such that B to C represents the time taken for the lowest SaO_2 in the lung at end apnea to be detected by an oximeter placed on the ear (ie, lung to ear circulation time). D is the end of the hyperpnea. Compared to the subject with idiopathic CSA (ICSA) shown in the lower panel, apnea duration (A to B) is similar (21 seconds), but lung to ear circulation time (B to C = 26 seconds), total cycle duration (A to D = 65 seconds), and hyperpnea duration (B to D = 46 seconds) are much longer. This is due to lower cardiac output in this patient since total cycle and hyperpnea durations, and lung to ear circulation time are inversely proportional to cardiac output. (*B*) Polysomnographic recording of a central apnea in a patient with ICSA. Note that compared to the patient with CSA-CSR in the upper panel, apnea length is similar (A to B = 18 seconds), but lung to ear circulation time (B to C = 8 seconds), total cycle duration (A to D = 25 seconds), and hyperpnea duration (B to D = 7 seconds) are much shorter. EEG, electroencephalogram; EKG, electrocardiogram, EMG_{at}, anterior tibialis electromyogram; EMG_{sm}, submental electromyogram; EOG, electrooculogram. (M J Hall, A Xie, R Rutherford, S Ando, J S Floras, T D Bradley, Cycle Length of Periodic Breathing in Patients With and Without Heart Failure, American Journal of Respiratory and Critical Care Medicine, 154 (2), August 1996, 376–381, https://doi.org/10.1164/ajrccm.154.2.8756809.)

have higher sympathetic nervous activity.[21] However, there is some evidence that the increased sympathetic activity related to CSA-CSR is due to more advanced HFrEF.[34] In a recent study, Horvath and colleagues[35] compared mortality rates among patients with HFrEF and either OSA or CSA-CSR, and found significantly higher mortality in those with CSA-CSR. However, those with CSA-CSR also had evidence of more advanced HFrEF including lower LVEF, more severe mitral regurgitation, higher rates of AF, and higher NT-proBNP concentrations. After controlling for these factors, there was no independent effect of CSA-CSR on mortality risk. Thus, although CSA-CSR may be a marker of higher mortality risk, this may be because it is also a marker of more severe HFrEF. However, a limitation of that study is that it did not include patients with HFrEF but without SDB.

TREATMENT

Optimization of Heart Failure Therapy

Since CSA-CSR is related to HFrEF severity, the initial management of CSA-CSR in patients with HFrEF should focus on optimization of the HF therapy itself. Contemporary HF therapy, including medications, cardiac resynchronization therapy, and exercise rehabilitation, may reduce the severity of CSA and CSA-CSR by reducing peripheral and pulmonary edema, and overnight rostral fluid shift as well as improving hemodynamic status with reduced circulation time.[36–40]

Supplemental Oxygen

Supplemental O_2 may reduce ventilatory instability and central respiratory events by attenuating hypoxic chemoreflex activation and decreasing loop gain.[41] The Impact of Low Flow Nocturnal Oxygen Therapy on Hospital Admissions and Mortality in Patients with HF and CSA (LOFT-HF) tested the hypothesis that supplemental O_2 at 3 L/min during sleep would reduce the primary composite endpoint of all-cause mortality, a life-saving cardiovascular intervention, cardiac transplantation, or unplanned hospitalization for worsening HF compared to sham O_2.[42] The estimated sample size was 858 patients with HFrEF and CSA-CSR. However, the trial was terminated after only 98 patients were enrolled and was underpowered to test the original hypothesis. O_2 reduced the AHI by only approximately 50%. There was a tendency to a higher primary even rate in the O_2 versus sham O_2 cohort (hazard ratio [HR] 1.46 [95% confidence interval (CI): 0.65, 3.29]) with no improvement in HF or sleep-related quality of life indices. The reason for lack of efficacy was not determined but one possibility is that supplemental O_2 in such patients caused hyperoxia and its adverse hemodynamic effects related to oxidative stress, such as raising vascular resistance, blood pressure and left ventricular (LV) filling pressure, and lowering cardiac output.[43,44] Taken together, there is insufficient evidence to support the use of O_2 to treat CSR-CSA in patients with HFrEF, and indeed, one must consider the possibility that supplemental O_2 may actually be harmful.

Respiratory Stimulants

Acetazolamide, a carbonic anhydrase inhibitor, induces a mild metabolic acidosis, thereby increasing ventilatory drive and widening the margin between resting $Paco_2$ and the apneic threshold. Javaheri and colleagues demonstrated in patients with HFrEF and CSA-CSR, that through this mechanism, it improved respiratory control system stability and reduced the central AHI by about 50%.[45] However, this study had a small sample size and was of only 6-day duration so that long-term effects on CSA-CSR and clinical outcomes were not assessed. Because of this, the potential adverse long-term effects of metabolic acidosis and hypokalemia[46] that might precipitate arrhythmias, acetazolamide cannot be recommended for therapy of CSA-CSR in the setting of HFrEF.

Theophylline, an adenosine antagonist, stimulates central respiratory drive and augments cardiac contractility. In a 5-day randomized trial involving 15 patients with HFrEF and CSR-CSA, theophylline reduced the AHI but clinical outcomes were not assessed.[47] It must be kept in mind, however, that whereas theophylline was once used routinely for treatment of acute HF, its use for this purpose was abandoned because it increases the risk of cardiac arrhythmias and sudden death.[48] Consequently, theophylline cannot be recommended for therapy of CSR-CSA since its long-term safety and efficacy have not been demonstrated.

Inhalation of CO_2 or the addition of dead space raises $Paco_2$ above the apnea threshold and thereby abolishes CSR-CSA instantaneously in patients with HFrEF.[2] However, because there is no evidence of long-term clinical benefits, and because CO_2 increases sympathetic nervous activity and disrupts sleep,[49] it cannot be recommended for therapy of CSR-CSA.

Continuous Positive Airway Pressure

In small short-term trials involving patients with HFrEF and CSA-CSR, continuous positive airway pressure (CPAP) has been shown to augment cardiac output in those with elevated LV filling pressures, to reduce central AHI by about 50%, to improve autonomic function by reducing sympathetic and augmenting vagal activity and baroreflex sensitivity and improving LVEF.[50–53]

The Canadian Continuous Positive Airway Pressure for Patients with Central Sleep Apnea and Heart Failure (CANPAP) trial was the first large, long-term randomized trial to evaluate CPAP for treatment of CSA-CSR in patients with HFrEF.[54] It included 258 subjects, and although CPAP attenuated CSA-CSA by approximately 50%, improved nocturnal oxygenation, and modestly increased LVEF, reduced sympathetic activity and increased 6-minute walking distance, it had no significant effect on heart transplant-free survival or CV hospitalizations.

In a subsequent post hoc analysis of the CANPAP cohort, among those in whom CPAP reduced the AHI below 15 after 3 months, heart transplant-free survival was greater than in the control group and those in whom CPAP failed to reduce the AHI below 15.[55] These findings suggested the concept that effective suppression of CSA-CSR may be a key factor in improving CV outcomes in patients with HFrEF and CSA-CSR. Consequently, among patients with HFrEF and CSA-CSR, it would be reasonable to provide a trial of CPAP and repeat a PSG after 1 to 3 months while wearing CPAP. If the AHI falls below 15, then CPAP could be continued, but if it did not fall below 15, it should be stopped as it may worsen outcomes in those in whom it does not suppress CSA-CSR.

Adaptive Servo-Ventilation

Adaptive servo-ventilation (ASV) was initially developed specifically to alleviate CSA-CSR in patients with HFrEF through dynamic adjustment of inspiratory pressure support. In the initial version of ASV, pressure support was triggered by falls in minute ventilation (ASV_{MV}).[56] Among patients with HFrEF and CSA-CSR, ASV_{MV} was more effective in suppressing the central AHI than CPAP, BilevelPAP, and supplemental O_2.

The (Adaptive Servo-Ventilation for Central Sleep Apnea in Systolic Heart Failure [SERVE-HF]) trial was the first large-scale, randomized trial designed to determine whether treatment of CSA-CSR with ASV_{MV} could improve cardiovascular outcomes in patients with HFrEF. Among 1325 participants, although ASV_{MV} effectively suppressed CSA, compared to the control group, it increased all-cause and cardiovascular mortality mainly due to an increase in sudden death (**Fig. 2**).[57] The cause of the increased sudden death rate was not identified.[58] It also had no beneficial effect on quality of

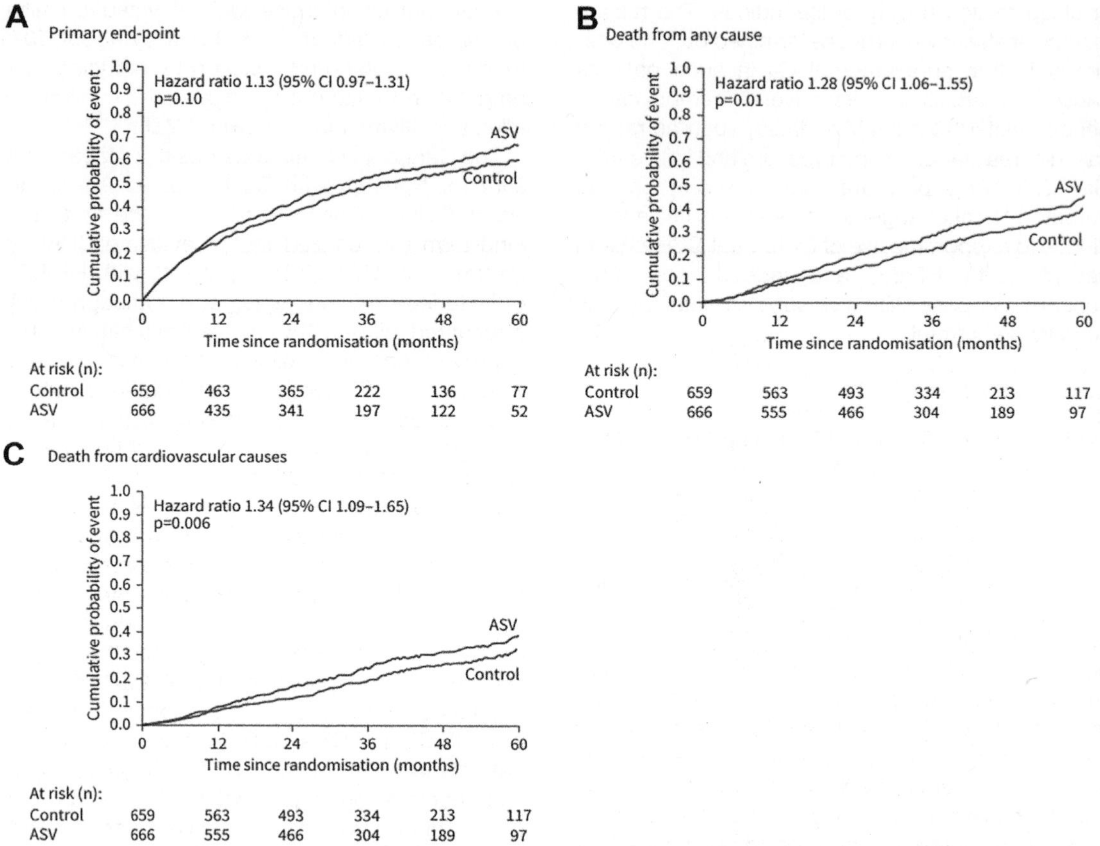

Fig. 2. (*A–C*) Effects of treating central sleep apnea in patients with heart failure and reduced ejection fraction by minute ventilation-triggered adaptive servo ventilation (ASV) in the SERVE-HF trial. Minute ventilation-triggered ASV had no effect on the primary endpoint, but increased both death from any cause and from cardiovascular causes. (From New England Journal of Medicine, Javaheri S et al., Effect of theophylline on sleep-disordered breathing in heart failure, 335 (8), 562-7. Copyright © 1996 Massachusetts Medical Society. Reprinted with permission from Massachusetts Medical Society.[47])

life assessed by the Minnesota Living with Heart Failure Questionnaire, New York Heart Association (NYHA) class or the Epworth Sleepiness Scale (ESS) score. These findings led to recommendations against ASV use in patients with HFrEF and predominantly CSA.[58,59]

Subsequent post hoc ancillary studies from the SERVE-HF trial reported that while ASV_{MV} reduced arousal frequency and stage N1 sleep time, it had no effect on stage N3 or REM sleep time.[60] ASV_{MV} also had no effect on echocardiographically assessed cardiac structure or function or biomarkers including NT-proBNP.[60,61] Because of the adverse effects of ASV_{MV} on mortality and absence of any significant symptomatic benefits in patients with HFrEF, this iteration of ASV_{MV} is no longer available for clinical use.

In patients with HFrEF and SDB, one type of apnea usually predominates at a single point in time.[6,12] If cardiac function changes, the predominant type can shift, in parallel: if OSA predominates, it can convert to CSA if HF worsens and vice versa, should it improve.[7,8,62] Accordingly, a newer version ASV, triggered by reductions in peak airflow (ASV_{PF}) was specifically designed to treat both CSA by automatically adjusting pressure support to treat central events, and unlike ASV_{MV}, by automatically adjusting end-expiratory pressure to treat obstructive events.[63] In a small-scale, short-term randomized trial, involving patients with HFrEF and coexisting OSA or CSA, Kasai and colleagues[63] tested the effects of ASV_{PF} compared to CPAP. Compared to CPAP, ASV_{PF} compliance was better; it was more effective in suppressing CSA-CSR and caused greater improvements in LVEF and quality of life.

The Adaptive Servo-ventilation for Sleep-disordered Breathing in Patients with Heart Failure with Reduced Ejection Fraction (ADVENT-HF) randomized trial evaluated the effects of ASV_{PF} on both OSA and CSA-CSR and on the primary composite endpoint of all-cause mortality, first admission to hospital for a cardiovascular reason, new onset AF or flutter requiring anticoagulation and delivery of an appropriate cardioverter-defibrillator shock.[6] It was stopped prematurely before reaching the estimated sample size of 860 because of COVID-19 restrictions on enrollment, and the Philips' recall of positive airway pressure devices for safety concerns related to potential disintegration of motor sound-abatement material.[64]

Seven hundred thirty-one patients were enrolled: 533 with predominantly OSA and 198 with predominantly CSA.[6] ASV_{PF} was very effective in controlling OSA and CSA such that it maintained the AHI in both groups below 5 throughout the maximum 5-year follow-up period. However, it had no significant effect on the primary endpoint either in the entire cohort or in the OSA or CSA cohorts (**Fig. 3**). However, in the CSA-CSR cohort, there was a trend to lower all-cause mortality among those randomized to ASV_{PF} (HR, 0.74, P = .25). Importantly, comparison of all-cause mortality hazard ratios between patients with CSA-CSR in SERVE-HF and ADVENT-HF reveals that the outcomes of ASV_{MV} and ASV_{PF} therapy, respectively, in the 2 trials were qualitatively and quantitatively different (HR 1.73; 95% CI: 1.00–2.99; P = .05; **Fig. 4**), consistent with the concept that these 2 devices behave differently in patients with HFrEF and CSA-CSR.[6,22] Similar to ASV_{MV} in SERVE-HF, ASV_{PF} in ADVENT-HF had no effect of LV structure of function.[65] However, in contrast to SERVE-HF, in ADVENT-HF, ASV_{PF} improved overall sleep structure with reduced arousal frequency and stage N1 sleep time and increased stage N3 and REM sleep time (**Table 1**).[6] It also improved MLHFQ and ESS

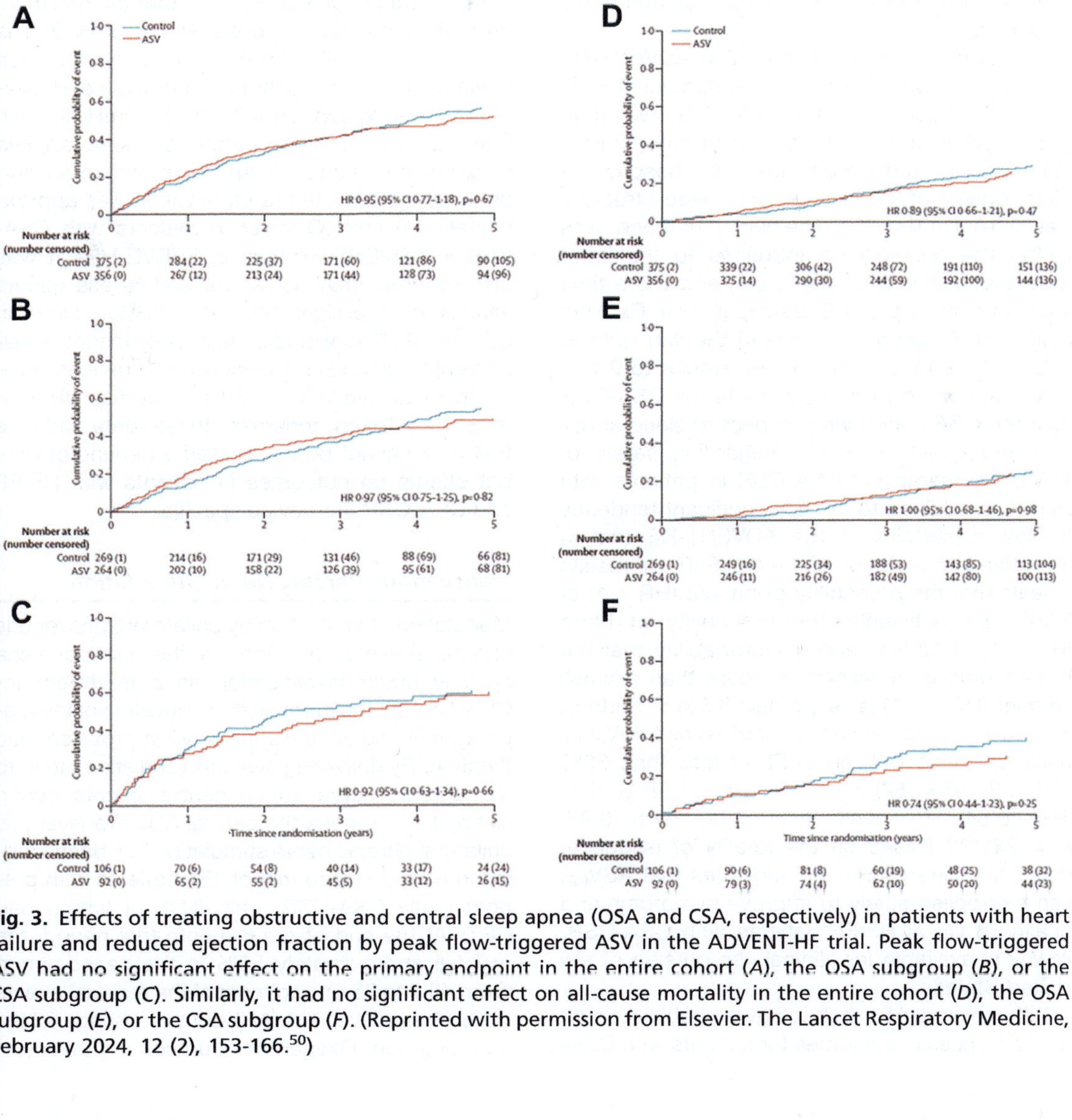

Fig. 3. Effects of treating obstructive and central sleep apnea (OSA and CSA, respectively) in patients with heart failure and reduced ejection fraction by peak flow-triggered ASV in the ADVENT-HF trial. Peak flow-triggered ASV had no significant effect on the primary endpoint in the entire cohort (*A*), the OSA subgroup (*B*), or the CSA subgroup (*C*). Similarly, it had no significant effect on all-cause mortality in the entire cohort (*D*), the OSA subgroup (*E*), or the CSA subgroup (*F*). (Reprinted with permission from Elsevier. The Lancet Respiratory Medicine, February 2024, 12 (2), 153-166.[50])

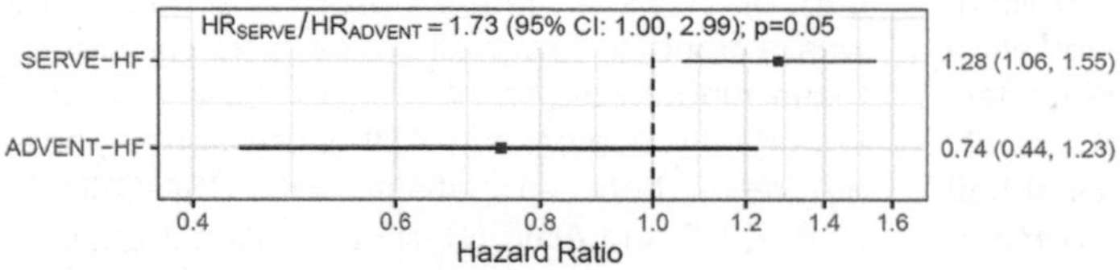

Fig. 4. Comparison of hazard ratios (HRs) for all-cause mortality in patients with CSA between minute ventilation triggered ASV in SERVE-HF and peak flow-triggered ASV in ADVENT-HF. The lower HR for peak flow-triggered ASV than for minute ventilation-triggered ASV, at a *P* value of 0.05, suggests qualitatively different effects with respect to this endpoint. (Reproduced with permission of the ERS 2026. Bradley TD, Logan AG, Floras JS. Treating sleep disordered breathing for cardiovascular outcomes: observational and randomised trial evidence. Eur Respir J 2024; 64: 2401033 [https://doi.org/10.1183/13993003.01033-2024].[7])

scores over the duration of the trial (**Fig. 5**) in the entire cohort, and in both the OSA and CSA cohorts. These data suggest that effects of interventions on symptoms and quality of life are related to effects on sleep structure rather than cardiac function. Thus, assessment of sleep structure while on SDB therapy may provide further insights into how various interventions affect symptomatic responses.

A win-ratio analysis incorporating ADVENT-HF clinical and patient-relevant endpoints favors overall ASV_{PF} treatment benefit. The win ratio calculated on sequential addition of outcomes to the hierarchy, in the order death, CV hospitalizations, quality of life indices, and sleep structure was 1.18 (1.00–1.39). The win difference was 7.6%. The principal contributions to the latter were better quality of life (4.2%) and more time spent in stage 3 plus REM sleep (2.1%). Ranking quality of life second increased the win ratio to 1.22 (1.04–1.43) and the win difference to 9.1%. ASV_{PF} appeared more effective in the CSA-CSR than the OSA cohort with respect to sleep structure and quality of life.[66] Regarding safety of ASV_{PF} for therapy of CSA-CSR in patients with HFrEF, in addition to the nonsignificant tendency for lower mortality in the ADVENT-HF trial, a Bayesian interpretation of the ADVENT-HF results reveals that the probability of benefit (HR $<$ 1) of 87.5% far outweighs the probability of harm (HR $>$ 1) of 12.5%, and the probability that the hazard ratio is increased by more than a small amount (HR $>$ 1.1) is very small: 6.5%.[67] Further, there was no difference in hazard ratios for ASV_{PF} between those with an LVEF of less than 30% (HR, 0.87; P = .52) and those with LVEF $\geqslant$ 30% (HR, 0.84; P = .45; interaction term 0.97, P = .93).[6,68] Based on the totality of evidence, data from the ADVENT-HF indicates that ASV_{PF}, can be applied safely to improve symptoms and quality of life in HFrEF patients with CSA-CSR. ASV_{PF} is available for clinical use outside of the United States.

Differences in ASV technology probably account for differences in outcomes for patients with CSA-CSR between SERVE-HF and ADVENT-HF. By automatically controlling pressure support and end-expiratory pressure, ASV_{PF} caused a greater reduction in AHI than ASV_{MV} probably by better controlling obstructive events.[6,58] The ASV_{MV} used in SERVE-HF had relatively high expiratory default settings of 5 cmH_2O and pressure support default settings of 3 cmH_2O, so that the minimum inspiratory pressure applied was 8 cmH_2O. The ASV_{PF} used in ADVENT-HF had a lower default minimum expiratory setting of 4 cmH_2O and minimum pressure support setting of 0 cmH_2O, such that the minimum inspiratory pressure applied would be only 4 cmH_2O. Applied pressure support up to 48 months after randomization was approximately 1.6 cmH_2O lower in patients with CSA-CSR in ADVENT-HF than in SERVE-HF.[6] It was also reported that ASV_{PF} generates less minute ventilation overnight than the ASV_{MV} used in SERVE-HF,[69] so would be less likely to induce hyperventilation and its adverse consequences, such as hypokalemia and malignant cardiac arrhythmias.[70,71] Taken together, these data indicate that ASV cannot be considered a generic device, but effects on outcomes in patients with HFrEF and CSA-CSR are device specific.

Transvenous Phrenic Nerve Stimulation

Modulation of ventilation by unilateral transvenous phrenic nerve stimulation via the superior vena cava is under investigation as a treatment for CSR-CSA on the premise that activation of the diaphragm during central apneas will improve cardiac function. By delivering synchronized stimulation to the phrenic nerve during central events during sleep, it can reduce the central AHI. Transvenous unilateral phrenic nerve stimulation has been studied in a randomized trial of 151 patients with predominantly CSA-CSR, only 64% of whom had HF.[72] At the end of the 6-month trial period, the AHI fell approximately 50% in the paced group (from 49.7 to 25.9), and most of the residual events were obstructive. The AHI did not change in the control group. Oxygen desaturation improved, as

Table 1
Effect of ASV_{PF} on polysomnographic variables from baseline to 1 month following randomization

	Control (n = 93)			ASV_{PF} (n = 84)			
Variable	**Baseline**	**1 mo**	**Difference**	**Baseline**	**1 mo**	**Difference**	***P***
AHI, events/h	50.6 ± 18.3	49.7 ± 23.5	−0.3 ± 20.9	50.5 ± 18.1	13.6 ± 12.2	−36.1 ± 18.7	<0.001
3% O_2 desaturation index, events/h	45.9 ± 19.8	43.8 ± 23.7	−1.5 ± 19.9	45.1 ± 18.2	10.4 ± 12.3	−34.3 ± 18.6	<0.001
Mean SaO_2, %	93.5 ± 2.4	93.7 ± 2.6	0.1 ± 1.6	93.5 ± 2.5	94.5 ± 2.1	1.0 ± 2.2	0.003
Min SaO_2, %	80.1 ± 10.0	80.4 ± 10.8	0.2 ± 7.5	78.8 ± 10.2	87.0 ± 4.8	7.8 ± 10.1	<0.001
Total sleep time, min	290.4 ± 72.0	299.8 ± 83.1	7.6 ± 74.9	286.2 ± 86.1	314.0 ± 86.3	24.6 ± 77.4	0.139
Sleep efficiency, %	67.5 ± 13.9	68.4 ± 16.1	0.8 ± 15.8	66.3 ± 18.5	72.5 ± 17.7	5.4 ± 16.2	0.054
Stage N1 sleep, min	52.0 ± 35.1	52.0 ± 34.9	−0.8 ± 29.9	46.0 ± 30.8	27.0 ± 21.3	−18.5 ± 33.0	<0.001
Stage N2 sleep, min	177.3 ± 56.4	182.2 ± 63.2	3.7 ± 61.7	181.7 ± 63.7	198.9 ± 62.1	13.2 ± 71.1	0.343
Stage N3 sleep, min	24.7 ± 22.9	24.3 ± 24.3	0.01 ± 24.0	24.3 ± 27.4	36.6 ± 29.0	12.2 ± 32.6	0.005
Stage REM sleep, min	36.9 ± 24.3	38.2 ± 26.4	0.9 ± 30.1	34.8 ± 24.8	47.7 ± 26.8	13.5 ± 25.2	0.003
Arousal index, events/h	45.4 ± 18.5	45.7 ± 21.6	0.2 ± 18.3	44.9 ± 21.3	24.9 ± 15.6	−19.3 ± 21.2	<0.001
PLM index, events/h	20.9 ± 30.3	21.7 ± 33.3	−0.2 ± 24.7	29.2 ± 34.9	43.2 ± 42.0	13.2 ± 29.3	0.001

Abbreviations: AHI, apnea-hypopnea index; ASV_{PF}, peak-flow-triggered adaptive servo-ventilation; PLM, periodic leg movements; REM, rapid eye movement; SaO_2, arterial oxyhemoglobin saturation.

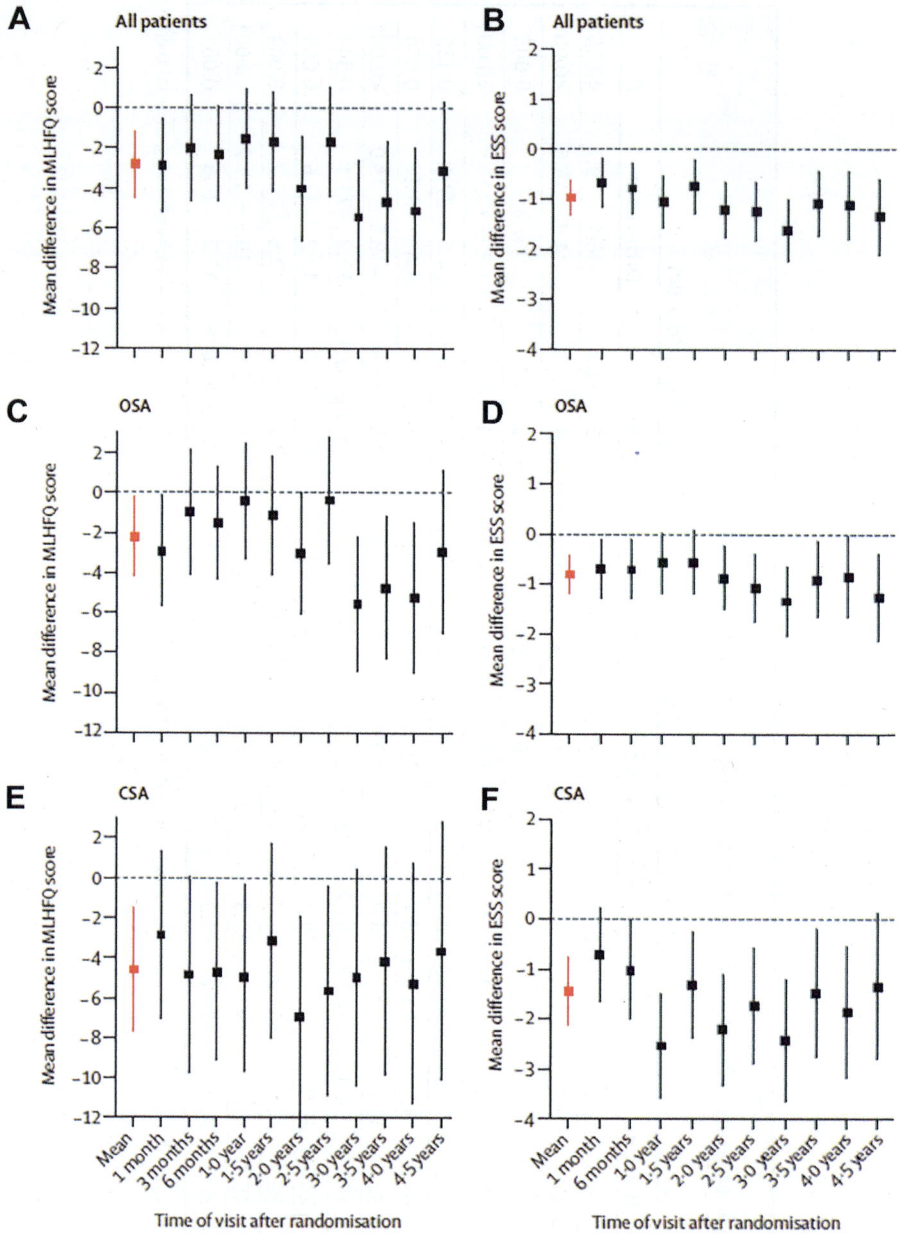

Number of assessments	1 month	1 year	2 years	3 years	4 years	1 month	1 year	2 years	3 years	4 years
Control	333	301	243	187	141	338	298	248	190	145
ASV	327	274	246	197	145	329	277	246	199	147

Fig. 5. (*A–F*) Effects of peak flow-triggered ASV on Minnesota Living with Heart Failure Questionnaire (MLHFQ) and Epworth Sleepiness Scale (ESS) from the ADVENT-HF trial. Differences in MLHFQ score and ESS scores between the peak-flow-triggered ASV and control groups. Over the entire trial period, the ASV_{PF} group had significant improvements in mean MLHFQ and ESS scores for the entire cohort (−2.8, 95% CI −1.2 to −4.5; P = .0009 and −1.0, 95% CI −0.6 to −1.3; P<.0001, respectively); the OSA subgroup (−2.2, −0.2 to −4.2; P = .028 and −0.8, −0.4 to −1.2; P = .0001, respectively), and the CSA subgroup (−4.6, −1.5 to −7.7; P = .0036 and −1.4, −0.8 to −2.1; P<.0001, respectively). (Reprinted with permission from Elsevier. The Lancet Respiratory Medicine, February 2024, 12 (2), 153-166.[50])

did daytime sleepiness and quality of life. The trial was not powered for cardiovascular events. The high residual AHI due mainly to obstructive events is a significant limitation in patients with HFrEF who often have combinations of CSA and OSA, and whose predominant type can change over time. It is possible phrenic nerve stimulation could induce upper airway obstruction due to asynchronous activation of the diaphragm and upper airway dilator muscles.[73] It is also possible that unilateral stimulation is not sufficient to abolish CSA-CSR in a substantial proportion of patients. In any case, further studies will be required to determine whether this therapy will improve cardiovascular outcomes.

Per cutaneous phrenic nerve stimulation was originally developed in 1948 to treat hypoventilation syndromes[74] and can be applied either unilaterally or bilaterally, safely over many years. Accordingly, it might be explored as an alternative to transvenous stimulation, as it is less invasive and can be applied bilaterally.

CENTRAL SLEEP APNEA IN ATRIAL FIBRILLATION

Epidemiology

Among patients with HFrEF, AF is associated with increased odds of having CSR-CSA.[2] Among patients with CSA but without HFrEF, cerebrovascular disease, or renal disease, AF was observed in 27%.[75] CSA is a predictor of incident AF risk in older men (>65 years).[76] Cross-sectional and observational studies suggest that CSA is more prevalent in patients with AF compared with those without AF.[75,76] The reason for the association between CSA and AF was not identified. However, the most likely possibility is that AF predisposes to CSA by mechanisms similar to those that predispose patients with HFrEF to CSR-CSA: AF lowers cardiac output and raises pulmonary venous pressure that could trigger hyperventilation and hypocapnia through stimulation of pulmonary vagal irritant receptors while recumbent during sleep.

Clinical Manifestations

Symptom profiles of CSA in patients with AF are not well described. It seems that CSA can present with nonspecific symptoms, including fatigue, and fragmented sleep.[75,77] Excessive daytime sleepiness is variably present and may be less prominent than expected relative to the degree of nocturnal respiratory instability, similar to that described for OSA in HFrEF.[19,20]

As a result, CSA may remain underdiagnosed in patients with AF unless actively screened using sleep studies. This underscores the importance of maintaining a high index of suspicion for CSA in AF populations, especially in the presence of HFrEF.

Prognostic Implications

The prognostic implications of CSA in patients with AF are unknown.

Treatment

In the absence of randomized trials of therapy of CSA in AF, management of CSA in patients with AF should primarily focus on optimization of AF treatment, including pharmacologic therapy, and radiofrequency ablation as required. A trial of CPAP or ASV_{PF} might be indicated if patients have symptomatic CSA. There is, however, no evidence that treating CSA in either paroxysmal or chronic AF will improve cardiovascular outcomes.

CENTRAL SLEEP APNEA IN CEREBROVASCULAR DISEASE

Epidemiology

SDB occurs in as many as 70% of patients after ischemic or hemorrhagic stroke.[78,79] OSA predominates, but CSA is also common. The prevalence appears to be highest in the acute post-stroke period, and severity of CSA tends to decrease over time.

The pathophysiology of CSA in the post-stroke period is poorly understood. However, in the subset with CSA-CSR, it is associated with occult LV dysfunction and hypocapnia.[80] This suggests that stroke per se may not be a cause of CSA-CSR, but that co-existing asymptomatic LV systolic dysfunction may be the culprit.

Clinical Manifestations

CSA in cerebrovascular disease may present with nocturnal periodic breathing, oxygen desaturation, sleep fragmentation, and reduced sleep efficiency. Daytime manifestations often overlap with post-stroke fatigue, cognitive impairment, and reduced vigilance, making clinical recognition challenging.[79]

Because these symptoms are frequently attributed to neurologic injury itself, CSA may be underrecognized unless polysomnography or respiratory monitoring is actively performed.[78] Also, CSA may dissipate over time for reason not well understood. This suggests that approaches to treatment need to take this time course into consideration and may require re-evaluation at regular intervals.

Prognostic Implications

A paucity of data on prognostic implications of CSA after stroke makes it difficult to determine its clinical significance. Prospective long-term studies would be required to shed light on this issue.

Treatment Considerations

Because of a lack of randomized clinical trials, indications for and treatment of CSA in cerebrovascular disease remains challenging. Optimization of underlying neurologic and cardiovascular status represents the primary therapeutic approach. In an observational study of 15 patients with CSA following stroke, ASV was found to be more effective than CPAP or bilevel-PAP in alleviating CSA. ASV caused a reduction in the AHI (46.7 $\pm$ 24.3 vs 8.5 $\pm$ 12/h, P = .001) and ESS score (8.7 $\pm$ 5.7 vs 5.6 $\pm$ 2.5, P = .08) with a mean nightly use of ASV of 5.4 $\pm$ 2.4 hours at 3 months after the initiation of treatment.[81] However, no randomized trials have assessed effects of treating CSA poststroke on long-term neurologic and functional outcomes.

SUMMARY

CSA and CSR are most common in the setting of HFrEF. So far, the best evidence for treatment indications comes for the ADVENT-HF trial, where ASV_{PF} alleviated CSA-CSR in association with improvements in HF and sleep apnea symptoms without causing either adverse or beneficial effects on morbidity or mortality. Thus, treatment of CSA-CSR in patients with HFrEF should be undertaken with the expectation of improvement in symptoms, but not cardiovascular endpoints. Long-term effects of phrenic pacing on cardiovascular outcomes remain to be determined. In the setting of AF and stroke, very little data are available on effects of treating CSA on clinical outcomes, such that treatment decisions need to be made on the basis of individual's symptoms and availability of therapeutic options. Close monitoring of symptoms in such cases is warranted. In general, more larger and longer-term randomized trials of treating CSA in the setting of AF and stroke are necessary to inform management decisions.

CLINICS CARE POINTS

- Treatment of CSR-CSA in patients with HFrEF should first involve optimization of heart failure therapy, but if CSR-CSA persists, ASVPF treatment can be applied to improve sleep quality and symptoms of heart faulure and sleep apnea.
- Treatment of CSA in AF should first involve optimization of AF therapy, but if CSA persists, ASV could be considered, but no randomized trials have demonstrated long-term beneficial effects of this or other interventions.
- For CSA following stroke, the possibility of underlying left venticular dysfunction should be investigated, and if found, treated. Otherwise, ASV could be applied for sleep apnea symptom relief, but without randomized trial evidence of benefit.

DISCLOSURE

S. Ishiwata received fellowship funding and T. D. Bradley received research grant support for the ADVENT-HF trial from Philips RS North America.

REFERENCES

1. Naughton M, Benard D, Tam A, et al. Role of hyperventilation in the pathogenesis of central sleep apneas in patients with congestive heart failure. Am Rev Respir Dis 1993;148(2):330–8.
2. Lorenzi-Filho G, Rankin F, Bies I, et al. Effects of inhaled carbon dioxide and oxygen on cheyne-stokes respiration in patients with heart failure. Am J Respir Crit Care Med 1999;159(5 Pt 1):1490–8.
3. Ryan CM, Bradley TD. Central sleep apnea, murray and nadel's textbook of respiratory medicine. 7th edition. Philadelphia (PA): Elsevier Saunders; 2021.
4. Sin DD, Fitzgerald F, Parker JD, et al. Risk factors for central and obstructive sleep apnea in 450 men and women with congestive heart failure. Am J Respir Crit Care Med 1999;160(4):1101–6.
5. Yumino D, Wang H, Floras JS, et al. Prevalence and physiological predictors of sleep apnea in patients with heart failure and systolic dysfunction. J Card Fail 2009;15(4):279–85.
6. Bradley TD, Logan AG, Lorenzi Filho G, et al, ADVENT-HF Investigators. Adaptive servo-ventilation for sleep-disordered breathing in patients with heart failure with reduced ejection fraction (ADVENT-HF): a multicentre, multinational, parallel-group, open-label, phase 3 randomised controlled trial. Lancet Respir Med 2024;12(2):153–66.
7. Tkacova R, Wang H, Bradley TD. Night-to-night alterations in sleep apnea type in patients with heart failure. J Sleep Res 2006;15(3):321–8.
8. Ryan CM, Floras JS, Logan AG, et al, CANPAP Investigators. Shift in sleep apnoea type in heart failure patients in the CANPAP trial. Eur Respir J 2010;35(3):592–7.
9. Lanfranchi PA, Braghiroli A, Bosimini E, et al. Prognostic value of nocturnal Cheyne-Stokes respiration in chronic heart failure. Circulation 1999;99(11):1435–40.
10. Bitter T, Faber L, Hering D, et al. Sleep-disordered breathing in heart failure with normal left ventricular ejection fraction. Eur J Heart Fail 2009;11(6):602–8.

11. Oldenburg O, Lamp B, Faber L, et al. Sleep-disordered breathing in patients with symptomatic heart failure: a contemporary study of prevalence in and characteristics of 700 patients. Eur J Heart Fail 2007;9(3):251–7.
12. Arzt M, Woehrle H, Oldenburg O, et al, SchlaHF Investigators. Prevalence and predictors of sleep-disordered breathing in patients with stable chronic heart failure: the SchlaHF registry. JACC Heart Fail 2016;4(2):116–25.
13. Borrelli C, Gentile F, Sciarrone P, et al. Central and obstructive apneas in heart failure with reduced, mid-range and preserved ejection fraction. Front Cardiovasc Med 2019;6:125.
14. Grimm C, Viniol C, Degerli M, et al. Sleep-disordered breathing in patients with heart failure with preserved left ventricular ejection fraction. Sleep Breath 2026;30(2).
15. Naughton MT. Cheyne-Stokes respiration: friend or foe? Thorax 2012;67(4):357–60.
16. Bradley TD, Phillipson EA. Central sleep apnea. Clin Chest Med 1992;13(3):493–505.
17. Yumino D, Bradley TD. Central sleep apnea and Cheyne-Stokes respiration. Proc Am Thorac Soc 2008;5(2):226–36.
18. Javaheri S. Sleep disorders in systolic heart failure: a prospective study of 100 male patients. The final report. Int J Cardiol 2006;106(1):21–8.
19. Taranto Montemurro L, Floras JS, Picton P, et al. Relationship of heart rate variability to sleepiness in patients with obstructive sleep apnea with and without heart failure. J Clin Sleep Med 2014;10(3):271–6.
20. Taranto Montemurro L, Floras JS, Millar PJ, et al. Inverse relationship of subjective daytime sleepiness to sympathetic activity in patients with heart failure and obstructive sleep apnea. Chest 2012;142(5):1222–8.
21. Spaak J, Egri ZJ, Kubo T, et al. Muscle sympathetic nerve activity during wakefulness in heart failure patients with and without sleep apnea. Hypertension 2005;46(6):1327–32.
22. Bradley TD, Logan AG, Floras JS. Treating sleep disordered breathing for cardiovascular outcomes: observational and randomised trial evidence. Eur Respir J 2024;64(6).
23. Berry RBBR, Gamaldo CE, et al. The AASM manual for the scoring of sleep and associated events: rules, terminology and technical specifications. 3 V, editor. Darien (IL): American Academy of Sleep Medicine; 2023.
24. Khoo MC, Kronauer RE, Strohl KP, et al. Factors inducing periodic breathing in humans: a general model. J Appl Physiol Respir Environ Exerc Physiol 1982;53(3):644–59.
25. Giannoni A, Gentile F, Navari A, et al. Contribution of the lung to the genesis of cheyne-stokes respiration in heart failure: plant gain beyond chemoreflex gain and circulation time. J Am Heart Assoc 2019;8(13):e012419.
26. Hall MJ, Xie A, Rutherford R, et al. Cycle length of periodic breathing in patients with and without heart failure. Am J Respir Crit Care Med 1996;154(2 Pt 1):376–81.
27. Redolfi S, Yumino D, Ruttanaumpawan P, et al. Relationship between overnight rostral fluid shift and Obstructive Sleep Apnea in nonobese men. Am J Respir Crit Care Med 2009;179(3):241–6.
28. Yumino D, Redolfi S, Ruttanaumpawan P, et al. Nocturnal rostral fluid shift: a unifying concept for the pathogenesis of obstructive and central sleep apnea in men with heart failure. Circulation 2010;121(14):1598–605.
29. Vazir A, Hastings PC, Papaioannou I, et al. Variation in severity and type of sleep-disordered breathing throughout 4 nights in patients with heart failure. Respir Med 2008;102(6):831–9.
30. Floras JS. Sleep apnea in heart failure: implications of sympathetic nervous system activation for disease progression and treatment. Curr Heart Fail Rep 2005;2(4):212–7.
31. Hanly PJ, Zuberi-Khokhar NS. Increased mortality associated with Cheyne-Stokes respiration in patients with congestive heart failure. Am J Respir Crit Care Med 1996;153(1):272–6.
32. Andreas S, Hagenah G, Moller C, et al. Cheyne-Stokes respiration and prognosis in congestive heart failure. Am J Cardiol 1996;78(11):1260–4.
33. Roebuck T, Solin P, Kaye DM, et al. Increased long-term mortality in heart failure due to sleep apnoea is not yet proven. Eur Respir J 2004;23(5):735–40.
34. Mansfield D, Kaye DM, Brunner La Rocca H, et al. Raised sympathetic nerve activity in heart failure and central sleep apnea is due to heart failure severity. Circulation 2003;107(10):1396–400.
35. Horvath CM, Floras JS, Yatsu S, et al. Event rates of patients with stable heart failure with reduced ejection fraction and newly diagnosed obstructive or central sleep apnoea. Eur J Heart Fail 2026;xuag110.
36. Bucca CB, Brussino L, Battisti A, et al. Diuretics in obstructive sleep apnea with diastolic heart failure. Chest 2007;132(2):440–6.
37. Tamura A, Kawano Y, Kadota J. Carvedilol reduces the severity of central sleep apnea in chronic heart failure. Circ J 2009;73(2):295–8.
38. Stanchina ML, Ellison K, Malhotra A, et al. The impact of cardiac resynchronization therapy on obstructive sleep apnea in heart failure patients: a pilot study. Chest 2007;132(2):433–9.
39. Oldenburg O, Faber L, Vogt J, et al. Influence of cardiac resynchronisation therapy on different types of sleep disordered breathing. Eur J Heart Fail 2007;9(8):820–6.

40. Yamamoto U, Mohri M, Shimada K, et al. Six-month aerobic exercise training ameliorates central sleep apnea in patients with chronic heart failure. J Card Fail 2007;13(10):825–9.
41. Franklin KA, Eriksson P, Sahlin C, et al. Reversal of central sleep apnea with oxygen. Chest 1997; 111(1):163–9.
42. Redline S, Li D, Javaheri S, et al. Nocturnal oxygen therapy for central sleep apnea in patients with heart failure: a multisite, double-blind, Sham-controlled randomized clinical trial (LOFT-HF). Ann Am Thorac Soc 2025;22(12):1951–60.
43. Haque WA, Boehmer J, Clemson BS, et al. Hemodynamic effects of supplemental oxygen administration in congestive heart failure. J Am Coll Cardiol 1996;27(2):353–7.
44. Mak S, Azevedo ER, Liu PP, et al. Effect of hyperoxia on left ventricular function and filling pressures in patients with and without congestive heart failure. Chest 2001;120(2):467–73.
45. Javaheri S. Acetazolamide improves central sleep apnea in heart failure: a double-blind, prospective study. Am J Respir Crit Care Med 2006;173(2): 234–7.
46. Wongboonsin J, Thongprayoon C, Bathini T, et al. Acetazolamide therapy in patients with heart failure: a meta-analysis. J Clin Med 2019;8(3).
47. Javaheri S, Parker TJ, Wexler L, et al. Effect of theophylline on sleep-disordered breathing in heart failure. N Engl J Med 1996;335(8):562–7.
48. Suissa S, Hemmelgarn B, Blais L, et al. Bronchodilators and acute cardiac death. Am J Respir Crit Care Med 1996;154(6 Pt 1):1598–602.
49. Andreas S, Weidel K, Hagenah G, et al. Treatment of Cheyne-Stokes respiration with nasal oxygen and carbon dioxide. Eur Respir J 1998;12(2): 414–9.
50. Kaneko Y, Floras JS, Usui K, et al. Cardiovascular effects of continuous positive airway pressure in patients with heart failure and obstructive sleep apnea. N Engl J Med 2003;348(13):1233–41.
51. Usui K, Bradley TD, Spaak J, et al. Inhibition of awake sympathetic nerve activity of heart failure patients with obstructive sleep apnea by nocturnal continuous positive airway pressure. J Am Coll Cardiol 2005;45(12):2008–11.
52. Gilman MP, Floras JS, Usui K, et al. Continuous positive airway pressure increases heart rate variability in heart failure patients with obstructive sleep apnoea. Clin Sci (Lond) 2008;114(3):243–9.
53. Ruttanaumpawan P, Gilman MP, Usui K, et al. Sustained effect of continuous positive airway pressure on baroreflex sensitivity in congestive heart failure patients with obstructive sleep apnea. J Hypertens 2008;26(6):1163–8.
54. Bradley TD, Logan AG, Kimoff RJ, et al, CANPAP Investigators. Continuous positive airway pressure for central sleep apnea and heart failure. N Engl J Med 2005;353(19):2025–33.
55. Arzt M, Floras JS, Logan AG, et al, CANPAP Investigators. Suppression of central sleep apnea by continuous positive airway pressure and transplant-free survival in heart failure: a post hoc analysis of the Canadian continuous positive airway pressure for patients with central sleep apnea and heart failure trial (CANPAP). Circulation 2007;115(25):3173–80.
56. Teschler H, Dohring J, Wang YM, et al. Adaptive pressure support servo-ventilation: a novel treatment for Cheyne-Stokes respiration in heart failure. Am J Respir Crit Care Med 2001;164(4):614–9.
57. Eulenburg C, Wegscheider K, Woehrle H, et al. Mechanisms underlying increased mortality risk in patients with heart failure and reduced ejection fraction randomly assigned to adaptive servoventilation in the SERVE-HF study: results of a secondary multistate modelling analysis. Lancet Respir Med 2016;4-(11):873–81.
58. Cowie MR, Woehrle H, Wegscheider K, et al. Adaptive servo-ventilation for central sleep apnea in systolic heart failure. N Engl J Med 2015;373(12): 1095–105.
59. ResMed Urgent Field Safety Notice. San Diego, CA, 2015.
60. Tamisier R, Pepin JL, Cowie MR, et al. Effect of adaptive servo ventilation on central sleep apnea and sleep structure in systolic heart failure patients: polysomnography data from the SERVE-HF major sub study. J Sleep Res 2022;31(6):e13694.
61. Cowie MR, Woehrle H, Wegscheider K, et al. Adaptive servo-ventilation for central sleep apnoea in systolic heart failure: results of the major substudy of SERVE-HF. Eur J Heart Fail 2018;20(3):536–44.
62. Tkacova R, Niroumand M, Lorenzi-Filho G, et al. Overnight shift from obstructive to central apneas in patients with heart failure: role of PCO2 and circulatory delay. Circulation 2001;103(2):238–43.
63. Kasai T, Usui Y, Yoshioka T, et al, JASV Investigators. Effect of flow-triggered adaptive servo-ventilation compared with continuous positive airway pressure in patients with chronic heart failure with coexisting obstructive sleep apnea and Cheyne-Stokes respiration. Circ Heart Fail 2010;3(1):140–8.
64. Philips. Voluntary Recall Information Philips Respironics Sleep and Respiratory Care devices. In: Philips, editor. June, 2021.
65. Yatsu S, Woo A, Horvath CM, et al, ADVENT-HF Investigators. LV structure and function in HFrEF with and without peak-flow-triggered adaptive servo-ventilation-treated sleep-disordered breathing. JACC Heart Fail 2026;14(2):102434.
66. Floras JS, Logan AG, Tomlinson G, et al. Win Ratio analysis for peak-flow adaptive servoventilation in treating sleep apnoea in heart failure with reduced ejection fraction. Can J Cardiol 2026.

67. Bradley TD, Logan AG, Tomlinson G, et al. Comment on ERS/ESRS statement on adaptive servo-ventilation for treatment of central sleep apnoea. Eur Respir J 2026;67(3).
68. Bradley TD, Logan AG, Lorenzi Filho G, et al. Supplement: adaptive servo-ventilation for sleep-disordered breathing in patients with heart failure with reduced ejection fraction (ADVENT-HF). Lancet Respir Med 2024.
69. Knitter J, Bailey OF, Poongkunran C, et al. Comparison of physiological performance of four adaptive servo ventilation devices in patients with complex sleep apnea. Am J Respir Crit Care Med 2019; 199(7):925–8.
70. Javaheri S, Shukla R, Wexler L. Association of smoking, sleep apnea, and plasma alkalosis with nocturnal ventricular arrhythmias in men with systolic heart failure. Chest 2012;141(6):1449–56.
71. Kulahcioglu S, Baysal PK, Kup A, et al. Bidirectional ventricular tachycardia induced by respiratory alkalosis mediated hypokalemia in a patient with acute ischemic heart failure. Pacing Clin Electrophysiol 2021;44(12):2115–8.
72. Costanzo MR, Ponikowski P, Coats A, et al. Phrenic nerve stimulation to treat patients with central sleep apnoea and heart failure. Eur J Heart Fail 2018;20-(12):1746–54.
73. Hyland RH, Hutcheon MA, Perl A, et al. Upper airway occlusion induced by diaphragm pacing for primary alveolar hypoventilation: implications for the pathogenesis of obstructive sleep apnea. Am Rev Respir Dis 1981;124(2):180–5.
74. Tibballs J. Diaphragmatic pacing: an alternative to long-term mechanical ventilation. Anaesth Intensive Care 1991;19(4):597–601.
75. Leung RS, Huber MA, Rogge T, et al. Association between atrial fibrillation and central sleep apnea. Sleep 2005;28(12):1543–6.
76. May AM, Blackwell T, Stone PH, et al, MrOS Sleep Outcomes of Sleep Disorders in Older Men Study Group. Central sleep-disordered breathing predicts incident atrial fibrillation in older men. Am J Respir Crit Care Med 2016;193(7):783–91.
77. Mehra R, Benjamin EJ, Shahar E, et al, Sleep Heart Health Study. Association of nocturnal arrhythmias with sleep-disordered breathing: the sleep heart health study. Am J Respir Crit Care Med 2006; 173(8):910–6.
78. Parra O, Arboix A, Bechich S, et al. Time course of sleep-related breathing disorders in first-ever stroke or transient ischemic attack. Am J Respir Crit Care Med 2000;161(2 Pt 1):375–80.
79. Kaneko Y, Hajek VE, Zivanovic V, et al. Relationship of sleep apnea to functional capacity and length of hospitalization following stroke. Sleep 2003;26(3): 293–7.
80. Nopmaneejumruslers C, Kaneko Y, Hajek V, et al. Cheyne-Stokes respiration in stroke: relationship to hypocapnia and occult cardiac dysfunction. Am J Respir Crit Care Med 2005; 171(9):1048–52.
81. Brill AK, Rosti R, Hefti JP, et al. Adaptive servo-ventilation as treatment of persistent central sleep apnea in post-acute ischemic stroke patients. Sleep Med 2014;15(11):1309–13.

Central Sleep Apnea in Renal and Endocrine Disease

Kimihiko Murase, MD, PhD[a], Owen D. Lyons, MBBChBAO, MCPI[b,c,d,e,*]

KEYWORDS

• Central sleep apnea • Chronic kidney disease • Hypervolemia • Acromegaly • Hypothyroidism

KEY POINTS

- Central sleep apnea (CSA) is prevalent, though often under-recognized, in conditions such as chronic kidney disease (CKD) and endocrine conditions such as acromegaly and hypothyroidism.
- End-stage renal disease (ESRD) is characterized by fluid overload predisposing to ventilatory control instability and CSA, while in acromegaly and hypothyroidism, changes in hormonal status can lead to direct effects on ventilatory control stability, predisposing to CSA.
- The presence of CSA in CKD may have a negative impact on kidney function mediated through the actions of intermittent hypoxia on the kidney medulla.
- In CKD and ESRD, optimization of fluid volumes through more intensified renal replacement therapy can attenuate CSA severity.
- In acromegaly and hypothyroidism, biochemical correction of the underlying hormonal imbalance can abolish CSA.

INTRODUCTION

Central sleep apnea (CSA) is a disorder characterized by a lack of drive to breathe during sleep. Rare in the general population, it is most commonly seen in patients with heart failure, but is also prevalent, though often under-recognized, in conditions such as chronic kidney disease (CKD), acromegaly and to a lesser extent hypothyroidism. CKD, especially end-stage renal disease (ESRD), similar to heart failure, is characterized by fluid overload, which can predispose to ventilatory control instability and subsequent development of CSA, while in endocrine diseases such as acromegaly and hypothyroidism, changes in hormonal and biochemical status can lead to direct effects on ventilatory control stability, predisposing to CSA. While there is a relative paucity of data compared to obstructive sleep apnea (OSA), there is evidence to suggest CSA may have an impact on morbidity and mortality in CKD, driven by the deleterious impact of intermittent hypoxia on kidney pathology. This article aims to review the prevalence, pathophysiology, diagnosis, and treatment of CSA in these disparate conditions.

DEFINITIONS AND DIAGNOSIS

CKD, defined by a glomerular filtration rate (GFR) less than 60 mL/minute/1.73 m^2 or the presence of pathologic evidence of kidney damage with a preserved GFR for $\geq$ 3 months.

ESRD, an advanced form of CKD, occurs when kidney function has deteriorated to an extent that

[a] Department of Advanced Medicine for Respiratory Failure, Kyoto University Graduate School of Medicine, Kyoto University, Kyoto, Japan; [b] Department of Medicine, University of Toronto, Toronto, Canada; [c] Department of Medicine, Women's College Hospital, Toronto, Canada; [d] Women's College Research Institute, Toronto, Canada; [e] Sleep Research Laboratory, KITE-UHN, Toronto, Canada
* Corresponding author. Division of Respirology, Women's College Hospital, 76 Grenville Street, Toronto, Ontario M5S 1B2, Canada.
E-mail address: owen.lyons@wchospital.ca

Sleep Med Clin 21 (2026) 333–341
https://doi.org/10.1016/j.jsmc.2026.05.003

Abbreviations	
AHI	apnea–hypopnea index
ASV	adaptive servo-ventilation
BPAP	bilevel positive airways pressure
CAPD	continuous ambulatory peritoneal dialysis
CHD	conventional hemodialysis
CKD	chronic kidney disease
CSA	central sleep apnea
ESRD	end-stage renal disease
GFR	glomerular filtration rate
GH	growth hormone
IGF-1	insulin-like growth factor-1
NHD	nocturnal hemodialysis
NPD	nocturnal peritoneal dialysis
ODI	oxygen desaturation index
OR	odds ratio
OSA	obstructive sleep apnea
PSG	polysomnography
RRT	renal replacement therapy

renal replacement therapy (RRT) in the form of chronic dialysis or transplant is required.

GFR, mathematically derived entity based on patient's serum creatinine, age, sex, and race, calculated by using one of several validated formulas.

Acromegaly, a rare disorder caused by the excessive production of growth hormone (GH), typically from a benign pituitary adenoma, after skeletal growth is complete. It results in the gradual enlargement of bones, cartilage, organs, and soft tissues, particularly in the hands, feet, and face.

Hypothyroidism, a disorder in which the thyroid gland does not produce sufficient thyroid hormones (T3 and T4), usually due to an issue with the thyroid gland itself or more rarely due to pituitary or hypothalamic failure.

Apnea, defined as the absence of tidal volume for at least 10 seconds. *Hypopnea,* defined as a decrease in the tidal volume of 30% for at least 10 seconds that is accompanied by at least a 3% decrease in oxygen saturation or is terminated by an arousal from sleep, as measured on overnight polysomnography (PSG).[1]

Obstructive or Central: Apneas are classified as obstructive if they are accompanied by inspiratory effort against the occluded pharynx, and central if they are not. Hypopneas are classified as obstructive if there are signs of upper airway flow limitation, or central if there are no such signs.

Apnea–hypopnea index (AHI), PSG measurement of sleep apnea severity. It is the average number of apneas and hypopneas per hour of sleep; sleep apnea can be classified as absent (AHI <5), mild (AHI 5–$<$ 15), moderate (AHI 15–$<$ 30) or severe (AHI ≥ 30).[2]

$PaCO_2$, the partial pressure of carbon dioxide in arterial blood.

Apnea threshold, the threshold level of $PaCO_2$ required to stimulate breathing.

CENTRAL SLEEP APNEA AND CHRONIC KIDNEY DISEASE

CKD is very common with 10% to 16% global prevalence.[3,4] Patients with CKD have increased morbidity and mortality, and this worsens as kidney function declines. ESRD in particular is associated with very high mortality, morbidity, and increased use of health care resources.[5,6] Compared to the general population, patients with CKD have a high prevalence of sleep-related breathing disorders including both OSA and CSA. In contrast to OSA which is characterized by repetitive pharyngeal collapse during sleep, CSA is characterized by a lack of drive to breathe during sleep,[7,8] with central apneas and hypopneas arising from complete or partial reductions in central neural outflow to the respiratory muscles during sleep.[1,2]

The presence of sleep apnea in CKD has been associated with poor sleep quality, poor quality of life, and increased cardiovascular risk, further contributing to the burden of heightened morbidity and mortality. However, although highly prevalent in CKD, sleep apnea, whether obstructive or central, remains under-recognized and under-diagnosed.

Prevalence, Presentation and Diagnosis of Central Sleep Apnea in Chronic Kidney Disease

There are several limitations in our understanding of true prevalence rates of CSA in CKD. Studies to date have been heterogenous in terms of the patient cohorts studied and also in the type of diagnostic tool used to diagnose sleep apnea, varying from in-lab PSG to a variety of different home sleep study diagnostic devices. Many research studies fail to differentiate between obstructive and CSA, instead using nonspecific terminology such as *sleep apnea* or *sleep-disordered breathing*. Further complicating this issue is that in patients with CKD there is significant night-to-night variability in both overall sleep apnea severity but also the predominant type of sleep apnea, obstructive or central, particularly in patients on dialysis, in whom there is marked night-to-night variability in fluid volume status. The implication of this is that a traditional one-night sleep study may not accurately capture the true burden of disease. It is estimated that compared to the general population, in which the prevalence of CSA is less than 1%, the prevalence of CSA is high in CKD is ~10%.[9,10] Furthermore, central events and mixed apneas are also commonly seen in CKD patients with predominantly obstructive events, and thus classified as OSA, and the prevalence rates of moderate–severe OSA in CKD range from 25% to 57% depending on the severity of the underlying kidney disease.[11–15] The increased prevalence of CSA in CKD is not explained by age or comorbidities, suggesting that the underlying kidney disease itself might be the main cause.[12,16,17]

The presence of CSA in CKD/ESRD is often not clinically apparent. Similar to heart failure patients with CSA, typical symptoms are of sleep fragmentation and daytime fatigue/tiredness rather than overt excessive sleepiness.[18,19] These symptoms are common and nonspecific in CKD patients, who often have other sleep disorders, such as restless legs syndrome and/or insomnia, which along with comorbid disease such as anemia and the underlying kidney disease itself, can lead to poor sleep and daytime tiredness, masking the presence of CSA.[20–22] It is not surprising therefore that there are no prediction scores or questionnaires to help identify the potential presence of CSA in CKD. Given the high prevalence of CSA and the fact it may not be clinically apparent, it has been suggested that diagnostic testing with overnight PSG should be considered in all patients with CKD, particularly in more advanced stages of disease.

Pathophysiology of Central Sleep Apnea in Chronic Kidney Disease

A growing body of evidence supports the concept of a bidirectional relationship between sleep apnea and CKD, in that the presence of OSA, and possibly CSA, can contribute to an accelerated decline in kidney function in patients with CKD, and in the later stages of disease, ESRD contributes to the pathogenesis of both OSA and CSA.

Central sleep apnea as a risk factor for worsening kidney function

There is a substantial body of evidence to support the role of OSA in accelerating decline in kidney function, through various pathophysiological mechanisms including intermittent hypoxia, increased negative intrathoracic pressure swings, and cortical arousals leading to sympathetic nervous system activation, hypertension, inflammation, oxidative stress and activation of the renin–angiotensin–aldosterone system.[23–30] CSA does not lead to increased negative intrathoracic pressure swings, given that central apneas/hypopneas occur in the presence of a patent airway, and is not associated with the same degree of cortical arousals as OSA, however, it does lead to intermittent hypoxia. While CSA is far less prevalent than OSA in the earlier stages of CKD, its presence can lead to worsening kidney function, mediated through intermittent hypoxia, which is of particular importance given the susceptibility of the kidney medulla to hypoxia.[23,31] While the kidneys receive about 25% of cardiac output, renal oxygen tension is relatively low due to low renal oxygen consumption. Intermittent hypoxia has been shown, in animal models of sleep apnea, to lead to kidney injury with histologic damage, characterized by glomerular hypertrophy, mesangial matrix expansion and increased cellular apoptosis.[32] Intermittent hypoxia has also been shown to activate the renin–angiotensin system in animal and human studies.[30,33,34] This in turn can lead to increased hypertension, hyperfiltration, and renal inflammation and fibrosis, leading to worsening CKD.[35]

In a prospective cross-sectional study of 7700 individuals from the European Sleep Apnea Database cohort the overnight minimum oxygen saturation was found to be an independent predictor of the presence of CKD, with a 2% higher probability of CKD for every unit decrease in the minimum oxygen saturation.[36] Another prospective study of more than 800 patients that followed changes in GFR over 2 years, of whom approximately 20% had CKD at baseline, showed that those with hypoxia (defined as ≥12% of the recording time with oxygen saturation <90%) had a higher risk (odds ratio [OR]) 2.89 (1.25–6.67) of rapid loss of kidney function (that is, estimated glomerular filtration rate [eGFR] decline ≥ 4/ml/minute/1.73 m^2 per year) after adjustment for sleep apnea severity and other recognized risk factors for CKD progression.[37] In a study of 161 patients with stage 3 to 4 CKD, GFR decline was 3- to 4-fold faster in patients with a 4% oxygen desaturation index (ODI) ≥15 compared with those with a 4% ODI less than 15, after adjustment for confounders.[38]

The role of chronic kidney disease/end-stage renal disease in the pathogenesis of central sleep apnea

Pathophysiological mechanisms related to the underlying CKD/ESRD that can lead to CSA include hypervolemia, altered chemosensitivity and possibly uremia-induced myopathy (**Fig. 1**).

While it has been postulated that uremia-induced neuropathy or myopathy may play a role in the pathogenies of both OSA and CSA, there are actually very little data regarding their role in the pathogenesis of CSA in ESRD. Uremic

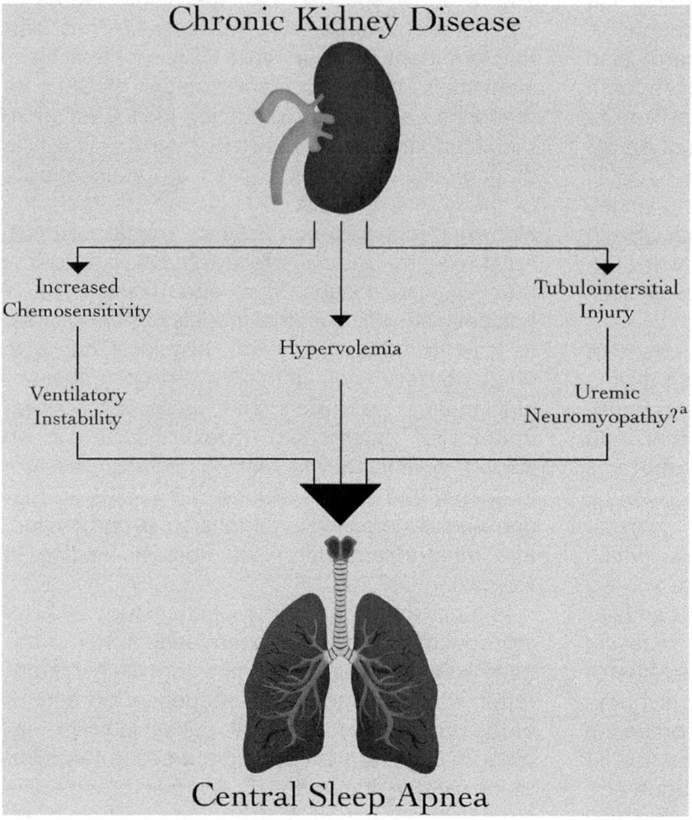

Fig. 1. Pathophysiological mechanisms promoting CSA in patients with ESRD. In CSA, the upper airway remains patent. ESRD-associated hypervolemia can lead to pulmonary congestion, similar to what is observed in heart failure, another condition in which CSA is common. This congestion leads to alterations in chemical feedback loop mechanisms to the respiratory center, which can in turn trigger cycles of hyperventilation alternating with central apneas or hypopneas. [a]While it has been postulated that uremic neuromyopathy may play a role in pathogenesis of sleep apnea, there is little data to support this.

myopathy increases fatigability of the respiratory muscles, including the diaphragm.[39] However, while this may contribute to a degree of hypoventilation it is not clear whether it leads to CSA and as such the concept of the role of uremic myopathy in the pathogenesis of CSA remains a hypothesis.

There is, however, a substantial body evidence to support the role of hypervolemia and altered chemosensitivity in the pathogenesis of both OSA and CSA in ESRD, similar to as in heart failure, which is also characterized by fluid overload and high prevalence of both types of sleep apnea.[40–42] Central apneas occur during sleep when the $PaCO_2$, decreases to less than the apnea threshold. Similar to heart failure patients with CSA who chronically hyperventilate causing hypocapnia with $PaCO_2$ closer to the apnea threshold than normal,[43,44] it has been shown that ESRD patients with CSA also have low-normal $PaCO_2$.[45] During sleep, any transient increase in ventilation for any reason, for example, an arousal, leads to a decrease in the $PaCO_2$ below the apnea threshold causing a central apnea. Fluid overload and nocturnal rostral fluid shift from the legs contributes to accumulation of fluid in the neck and chest.[40–42] Fluid accumulation in the lungs stimulates pulmonary irritant receptors causing chronic hyperventilation and leading to CSA by promoting cycles of hyperventilation and apnea,.[42,46]

The role of hypervolemia in the pathogenesis of CSA in CKD is supported by findings from observational studies. In a cross-sectional study of patients with CKD who were not receiving dialysis and had a body mass index of 24 $\pm$ 3.9 kg/m^2, brain natriuretic peptide levels and cardiothoracic ratio were significantly higher in those with severe sleep apnea than in those without sleep apnea.[47] Among patients with ESRD on conventional hemodialysis (CHD), those with moderate–severe sleep apnea had a greater total body extracellular fluid volume (>2 L) than those with mild or no sleep apnea and in a multivariate analysis, the total body extracellular fluid volume was the only factor that was independently and directly associated with sleep apnea severity (r = 0.47, *P* = .002).[12] Other studies have shown that interdialytic weight gain greater than 2 kg and the degree of fluid overload posthemodialysis are independent predictors of sleep apnea severity in patients with ESRD on CHD.[48,49] Increased ventilatory sensitivity to hypercapnia has also been shown to correlate with CSA severity in patients with ESRD.[50] Furthermore, transition from CHD to nocturnal hemodialysis (NHD) reduced ventilatory sensitivity, which was associated with a decrease in CSA severity.[51]

Impact of Central Sleep Apnea on Morbidity and Mortality in Chronic Kidney Disease/End-stage Renal Disease

The evidence base linking CSA with morbidity and mortality in CKD is quite limited.

One prospective study of 180 patients with CKD followed over 9 years, in whom just more than half had ESRD, showed that although sleep apnea severity, as measured by AHI, was not associated with increased mortality when adjusted for confounders, measures of overnight hypoxic burden—a higher proportion of sleep time with oxygen saturation less than 90% and lower mean oxygen saturation—were significantly associated with higher mortality hazard ratio (HR), 1.4; 95% confidence interval (CI), 1.1–1.7; $P = .007$ for every 15% higher proportion of time with low oxygen saturation, and HR, 1.6; 95% CI, 1.2–2.1; $P = .003$ for every 2% lower mean oxygen saturation).[52] In a recent large retrospective cohort study of the United States Renal Data system, of more than 600,000 patients, the presence of CSA was associated with an increased risk of stroke (adjusted relative risk [aRR] 1.69, 95% CI = 1.28–2.23) and increased mortality (adjusted hazard ratio [aHR] 1.42, 95% CI 1.29–1.56) thought the methodology likely led to under-recognition of the presence of CSA with a reported prevalence of only 0.1%.[53,54]

Treatment of Central Sleep Apnea in Chronic Kidney Disease

Positive airway pressure (PAP) therapy for central sleep apnea in chronic kidney disease

There is a paucity of evidence-based guidelines to inform treatment of CSA in CKD or ESRD. A meta-analysis of 8 studies, that included patients with both OSA and CSA, treated with continuous positive airway pressure (CPAP), bilevel positive airways pressure (BPAP) or adaptive servo-ventilation (ASV) showed no overall change in GFR before and after PAP treatment in patients with sleep apnea.[55] However, in a subgroup analysis of the data, longer PAP usage duration and increased age were associated with significant improvements in GFR.[55] There are no CKD-specific data to guide treatment of CSA for subjective improvement in terms of sleep quality or overall quality of life. Recent 2025 American Academy of Sleep Medicine (AASM) guidelines on treatment of CSA reflect the lack of evidence, with conditional recommendations based on low certainty evidence for the use of CPAP or ASV for treatment of CSA in CKD, and conditional recommendation based on very low certainty evidence for BPAP with a backup rate.[56] PAP therapy can be challenging in all patients but can be particularly so in CKD and especially ESRD patients given the burden of their underlying kidney disease, the burden of treatment, and the impact of comorbidities including other sleep disorders such as restless leg syndrome and insomnia.[22]

Impact of intensification of renal replacement therapy on central sleep apnea severity

A meta-analysis of 9 studies that evaluated the impact of RRT modality on sleep apnea severity showed that intensive RRT was superior to conventional RRT in AHI reduction (OR 0.66, CI 95% 0.51–0.84, $P<.001$) and sleep quality improvement.[57] In patients with ESRD, intensification of dialysis treatment, either by conversion from CHD to NHD, or from continuous ambulatory peritoneal dialysis (CAPD) to nocturnal peritoneal dialysis (NPD), has been shown to reduce sleep apnea severity.[58,59] In a study of 14 patients with ESRD on thrice-weekly CHD, conversion to NHD reduced AHI from 25 $\pm$25 to 8$\pm$8 ($P = .03$).[58] While fluid volumes were not measured in this study, a more recent study evaluated the impact of fluid removal on sleep apnea severity using ultrafiltration. The study included 15 individuals on CHD with moderate–severe sleep apnea (including OSA and CSA) and showed a 36% reduction in AHI after fluid removal during a single ultrafiltration session with average volume removed of 2.2 L. Uremic and metabolic status were unchanged.[45] In those subjects with CSA, the AHI decreased by 40% from 60.4 $\pm$ 16.7 to 36.0 $\pm$ 19.1 ($P = .003$). The study also showed a correlation between AHI reduction and the decrease in total body fluid volume ($r = 0.567$; $P = .027$) and a reduction in thoracic fluid volume of approximately 500 mL ($P<.001$) postultrafiltration as measured by bioelectrical impedance. Furthermore transcutaneous CO_2 levels also normalized with the decrease in fluid volume, suggesting a decrease in respiratory drive and possibly improved ventilatory stability.[45] In a study of patients with ESRD on CAPD, conversion to NPD led to a reduction in prevalence of sleep apnea from 33.3% to 4.2%, in association with a reduction in total body water from 35.1 $\pm$ 7.35 L to 32.8 $\pm$ 7.37 ($P = .004$), further highlighting the important role of hypervolemia in the pathogenesis of sleep apnea ESRD.

Summary

CSA is far more common in CKD than the general population and its presence has potential significant impact for morbidity and mortality, mediated through intermittent hypoxia. As CKD progresses, CSA is even more common, underpinning the concept of a bidirectional relationship between the disorders, with hypervolemia playing an important role in CSA pathogenesis. Given the increased prevalence of CSA in CKD and its potential impact on outcomes, there should be a low threshold to proceed with diagnostic testing for CSA in this population. While PAP therapy still plays an important role in terms of treatment options there are practical barriers to adherence. Optimization of fluid volume status by conversion to NHD or NPD can attenuate sleep apnea severity, in some cases obviating the need for PAP therapy.

CENTRAL SLEEP APNEA AND HYPOTHYROIDISM

Hypothyroidism is a relatively common endocrine disorder with prevalence rates of biochemical (subclinical) hypothyroidism occurring in 4% to 5% of the population, with overt clinical hypothyroidism occurring in 0.3%–0.4%.[60] It is a disorder in which the thyroid gland does not produce sufficient thyroid hormones (T3 and T4), usually due to an issue with the thyroid gland itself or more rarely due to pituitary or hypothalamic failure. OSA occurs in approximately 20% to 25% of patients with hypothyroidism, thought to be possibly due to narrowing of the upper airway secondary to deposition of mucopolysaccharides and protein extravasation into the tissues, while CSA is far less common and is associated with more severe cases, which were more common historically than currently.[61,62]

Thyroid hormones are important to ensure normal sensitivity of chemoreceptors and deficiency of thyroid hormones may manifest with blunted ventilatory responses, with subsequent correction of the deficiency with exogenous thyroxine leading to normalization of the ventilatory response and attenuation of CSA severity.[61–63] Interestingly, women seem to be more vulnerable to the effect of hypothyroidism on ventilatory drive.[62]

CENTRAL SLEEP APNEA AND ACROMEGALY

Acromegaly is a rare endocrine disorder, with reported prevalence of 122 cases/10^6 persons. It is caused by excessive secretion of GH and insulin-like growth factor-1 (IGF-1), usually from a benign pituitary hormone[64] and results in the gradual enlargement of bones, cartilage, organs, and soft tissues, particularly in the hands, feet, and face. Soft tissue hypertrophy in the upper airway can lead to OSA, and the prevalence of OSA is reported to be as high as 60%.[65–67] Interestingly, CSA, though less common than OSA, is prevalent and has been reported to occur in 5% to 10% of cases.[68] It is has been shown that acromegalic patients with CSA have increased GH and IGF-1 levels compared with their counterparts with OSA.[68] Furthermore, measures of ventilatory responsiveness correlate with GH levels.[68] It is thought that GH and IGF-1 directly sensitize the central chemoreceptors leading to ventilatory instability. Identification of CSA in patients with acromegaly is important as it is a condition associated with increased cardiovascular risk of hypertension, arrythmias and cardiomyopathy. Biochemical control of acromegaly with either surgical resection or somatostatin analogs may lead to a reduction in CSA severity. If there is persistence of CSA, PAP therapy with CPAP or ASV can be used.[56]

SUMMARY

CSA is often under-recognized in endocrine conditions such as acromegaly and hypothyroidism. In both conditions, hormonal changes seem to play a role in leading to ventilatory instability and subsequent CSA. While relatively rare, the presence of CSA is associated with poorer outcomes in these conditions. While biochemical correction of the underlying hormonal imbalance with surgery or medication often leads to a resolution of CSA, PAP therapy can be considered if CSA persists.

CLINICS CARE POINTS

- Given the increased prevalence of CSA in CKD and its potential impact on morbidity and mortality, clinicians should have a low threshold for screening for its presence.
- PAP therapy plays an important role in treatment of CSA but in patients with CKD/ESRD, adherence to treatment can be a problem due to the impact of co-morbid disease, insomnia and other factors.
- Before considering PAP therapy for treatment of CSA in ESRD, consideration should be given to optimization of fluid volume status by intensification of dialysis, which may obviate the need for PAP therapy.
- While CSA is rare in endocrine diseases, clinicians should be aware that its presence can be associated with increased mortality.

REFERENCES

1. Berry RB, Brooks R, Gamaldo CE, et al, for the American Academy of Sleep Medicine. The AASM manual for the scoring of sleep and associated events: rules, terminology and technical specifications. Version 2.4, 2017, American Academy of Sleep Medicine. J Clin Sleep Med 2017;13(5):665–6.
2. AASM. Sleep-related breathing disorders in adults: recommendations for syndrome definition and measurement techniques in clinical research. The report of an American academy of sleep medicine task force. Sleep 1999;22:667–89. https://doi.org/10.1378/chest.97.1.27.
3. Jha V, Garcia-Garcia G, Iseki K, et al. Chronic kidney disease: global dimension and perspectives. Lancet (London, England) 2013;382:260–72.
4. Xie Y, Bowe B, Mokdad AH, et al. Analysis of the Global Burden of Disease study highlights the global, regional, and national trends of chronic kidney disease epidemiology from 1990 to 2016. Kidney Int 2018;94:567–81.
5. Daratha KB, Short RA, Corbett CF, et al. Risks of subsequent hospitalization and death in patients with kidney disease. Clin J Am Soc Nephrol 2012; 7:409–16.
6. Klarenbach SW, Tonelli M, Chui B, et al. Economic evaluation of dialysis therapies. Nat Rev Nephrol 2014;10:644–52.
7. Yumino D, Bradley TD. Central sleep apnea and Cheyne-Stokes respiration. Proc Am Thorac Soc 2008;5:226–36.
8. Jordan AS, McSharry DG, Malhotra A. Adult obstructive sleep apnoea. Lancet (London, England) 2014; 383:736–47.
9. Donovan LM, Kapur VK. Prevalence and characteristics of central compared to obstructive sleep apnea: analyses from the sleep heart health study cohort. Sleep 2016;39:1353–9.
10. Nigam G, Pathak C, Riaz M. A systematic review of central sleep apnea in adult patients with chronic kidney disease. Sleep Breath 2016;20:957–64.
11. Nicholl DDM, Ahmed SB, Loewen AHS, et al. Declining kidney function increases the prevalence of sleep apnea and nocturnal hypoxia. Chest 2012; 141:1422–30.
12. Lyons OD, Inami T, Perger E, et al. The effect of fluid overload on sleep apnoea severity in haemodialysis patients. Eur Respir J 2017;49:1601789. https://doi.org/10.1183/13993003.01789-2016.
13. Roumelioti ME, Buysse DJ, Sanders MH, et al. Sleep-disordered breathing and excessive daytime sleepiness in chronic kidney disease and hemodialysis. Clin J Am Soc Nephrol 2011;6:986–94.
14. Markou N, Kanakaki M, Myrianthefs P, et al. Sleep-disordered breathing in nondialyzed patients with chronic renal failure. Lung 2006;184:43–9.
15. Sakaguchi Y, Shoji T, Kawabata H, et al. High prevalence of obstructive sleep apnea and its association with renal function among nondialysis chronic kidney disease patients in Japan: a cross-sectional study. Clin J Am Soc Nephrol 2011;6: 995–1000.
16. Unruh ML, Sanders MH, Redline S, et al. Sleep apnea in patients on conventional thrice-weekly hemodialysis: Comparison with matched controls from the sleep heart health study. J Am Soc Nephrol 2006;17: 3503–9.
17. Beecroft JM, Pierratos A, Hanly PJ. Clinical presentation of obstructive sleep apnea in patients with end-stage renal disease. J Clin Sleep Med 2009;5: 115–21.
18. Javaheri S, Parker TJ, Liming JD, et al. Sleep apnea in 81 ambulatory male patients with stable heart failure. Types and their prevalences, consequences, and presentations. Circulation 1998;97:2154–9.
19. Bradley TD, Floras JS. Sleep apnea and heart failure: part II: central sleep apnea. Circulation 2003; 107:1822–6.
20. Sekercioglu N, Curtis B, Murphy S, et al. Sleep quality and its correlates in patients with chronic kidney disease: a cross-sectional design. Ren Fail 2015; 37:757–62.
21. Unruh ML, Hartunian MG, Chapman MM, et al. Sleep quality and clinical correlates in patients on maintenance dialysis. Clin Nephrol 2003;59:280–8.
22. Lyons OD. Sleep disorders in chronic kidney disease. Nat Rev Nephrol 2024;20:690–700.
23. Sun W, Yin X, Wang Y, et al. Intermittent hypoxia-induced renal antioxidants and oxidative damage in male mice: hormetic dose response. Dose Response 2012;11:385–400.
24. Brooks D, Horner RL, Kozar LF, et al. Obstructive sleep apnea as a cause of systemic hypertension. Evidence from a canine model. J Clin Investig 1997;99: 106–9.
25. Horner RL, Brooks D, Kozar LF, et al. Immediate effects of arousal from sleep on cardiac autonomic outflow in the absence of breathing in dogs. J Appl Physiol 1995;79:151–62.
26. Somers VK, Dyken ME, Clary MP, et al. Sympathetic neural mechanisms in obstructive sleep apnea. J Clin Investig 1995;96:1897–904.
27. Yokoe T, Minoguchi K, Matsuo H, et al. Elevated levels of C-reactive protein and interleukin-6 in patients with obstructive sleep apnea syndrome are decreased by nasal continuous positive airway pressure. Circulation 2003;107:1129–34.
28. Ryan S, Taylor CT, McNicholas WT. Selective activation of inflammatory pathways by intermittent hypoxia in obstructive sleep apnea syndrome. Circulation 2005;112:2660–7.
29. Dyugovskaya L, Lavie P, Lavie L. Increased adhesion molecules expression and production of reactive

oxygen species in leukocytes of sleep apnea patients. Am J Respir Crit Care Med 2002;165:934–9.
30. Zalucky AA, Nicholl DDM, Hanly PJ, et al. Nocturnal hypoxemia severity and renin-angiotensin system activity in obstructive sleep apnea. Am J Respir Crit Care Med 2015;192:873–80.
31. Evans RG, Goddard D, Eppel GA, et al. Factors that render the kidney susceptible to tissue hypoxia in hypoxemia. Am J Physiol Regul Integr Comp Physiol 2011;300:R931–40.
32. Abuyassin B, Badran M, Ayas NT, et al. Intermittent hypoxia causes histological kidney damage and increases growth factor expression in a mouse model of obstructive sleep apnea. PLoS One 2018;13: e0192084. https://doi.org/10.1371/journal.pone.0192084.
33. Fletcher EC, Bao G, Li R. Renin activity and blood pressure in response to chronic episodic hypoxia. Hypertension 1999;34:309–14.
34. Foster GE, Hanly PJ, Ahmed SB, et al. Intermittent hypoxia increases arterial blood pressure in humans through a Renin-Angiotensin system-dependent mechanism. Hypertension 2010;56:369–77.
35. Hanly PJ, Ahmed SB. Sleep apnea and the kidney: is sleep apnea a risk factor for chronic kidney disease? Chest 2014;146:1114–22.
36. Marrone O, Battaglia S, Steiropoulos P, et al. Chronic kidney disease in European patients with obstructive sleep apnea: the ESADA cohort study. J Sleep Res 2016;25:739–45.
37. Ahmed SB, Ronksley PE, Hemmelgarn BR, et al. Nocturnal hypoxia and loss of kidney function. PLoS One 2011;6:e19029. https://doi.org/10.1371/journal.pone.0019029.
38. Sakaguchi Y, Hatta T, Hayashi T, et al. Association of nocturnal hypoxemia with progression of CKD. Clin J Am Soc Nephrol 2013;8:1502–7.
39. Tarasuik A, Heimer D, Bark H. Effect of chronic renal failure on skeletal and diaphragmatic muscle contraction. Am Rev Respir Dis 1992;146:1383–8.
40. Elias RM, Chan CT, Paul N, et al. Relationship of pharyngeal water content and jugular volume with severity of obstructive sleep apnea in renal failure. Nephrol Dial Transplant 2013;28:937–44.
41. Elias RM, Bradley TD, Kasai T, et al. Rostral overnight fluid shift in end-stage renal disease: relationship with obstructive sleep apnea. Nephrol Dial Transplant 2012;27:1569–73.
42. Yumino D, Redolfi S, Ruttanaumpawan P, et al. Nocturnal rostral fluid shift: a unifying concept for the pathogenesis of obstructive and central sleep apnea in men with heart failure. Circulation 2010; 121:1598–605.
43. Naughton M, Benard D, Tam A, et al. Role of hyperventilation in the pathogenesis of central sleep apneas in patients with congestive heart failure. Am Rev Respir Dis 1993;148:330–8.
44. Hanly P, Zuberi N, Gray R. Pathogenesis of Cheyne-Stokes respiration in patients with congestive heart failure. Relationship to arterial PCO2. Chest 1993; 104:1079–84.
45. Lyons OD, Chan CT, Yadollahi A, et al. Effect of ultrafiltration on sleep apnea and sleep structure in patients with end-stage renal disease. Am J Respir Crit Care Med 2015;191:1287–94.
46. Anastassov GE, Trieger N. Edema in the upper airway in patients with obstructive sleep apnea syndrome. Oral Surg Oral Med Oral Pathol Oral Radiol Endod 1998;86:644–7.
47. Tanaka A, Inaguma D, Ito E, et al. Factors associated with severity of sleep apnoea syndrome in patients with chronic kidney disease. Acta Cardiol 2017;72:440–5.
48. Harmon RR, De Lima JJG, Drager LF, et al. Obstructive sleep apnea is associated with interdialytic weight gain and increased long-term cardiovascular events in hemodialysis patients. Sleep Breath 2018; 22:721–8.
49. Ogna A, Forni Ogna V, Mihalache A, et al. Obstructive sleep apnea severity and overnight body fluid shift before and after hemodialysis. Clin J Am Soc Nephrol 2015;10:1002–10.
50. Beecroft J, Duffin J, Pierratos A, et al. Enhanced chemo-responsiveness in patients with sleep apnoea and end-stage renal disease. Eur Respir J 2006;28: 151–8.
51. Beecroft JM, Duffin J, Pierratos A, et al. Decreased chemosensitivity and improvement of sleep apnea by nocturnal hemodialysis. Sleep Med 2009;10: 47–54.
52. Jhamb M, Ran X, Abdalla H, et al. Association of sleep apnea with mortality in patients with advanced kidney disease. Clin J Am Soc Nephrol 2020;15: 182–90.
53. Acree L, Waller J, Bollag W, et al. Sleep apnea in end-stage renal disease patients: impact on cardiovascular and neurological outcomes. J Postgrad Med 2024;70:36–42.
54. Prabu P, Acree L, Waller JL, et al. Sleep apnea in end-stage renal disease patients: risk factors and mortality. J Investig Med 2023;71:465–70.
55. Chen LD, Lin L, Ou YW, et al. Effect of positive airway pressure on glomerular filtration rate in patients with sleep-disordered breathing: a meta-analysis. Sleep Breath 2017;21:53–9.
56. Badr MS, Khayat RN, Allam JS, et al. Treatment of central sleep apnea in adults: an American Academy of Sleep Medicine clinical practice guideline. J Clin Sleep Med 2025;21:2181–91.
57. Kennedy C, Ryan SA, Kane T, et al. The impact of change of renal replacement therapy modality on sleep quality in patients with end-stage renal disease: a systematic review and meta-analysis. J Nephrol 2018;31:61–70.

58. Hanly PJ, Pierratos A. Improvement of sleep apnea in patients with chronic renal failure who undergo nocturnal hemodialysis. N Engl J Med 2001;344: 102–7.
59. Tang SC, Lam B, Ku PP, et al. Alleviation of sleep apnea in patients with chronic renal failure by nocturnal cycler-assisted peritoneal dialysis compared with conventional continuous ambulatory peritoneal dialysis. J Am Soc Nephrol 2006;17:2607–16.
60. Wyne KL, Nair L, Schneiderman CP, et al. Hypothyroidism prevalence in the United States: a retrospective study combining national health and nutrition examination survey and claims data, 2009-2019. J Endocr Soc 2022;7:bvac172. https://doi.org/10.1210/jendso/bvac172.
61. Millman RP, Bevilacqua J, Peterson DD, et al. Central sleep apnea in hypothyroidism. Am Rev Respir Dis 1983;127:504–7.
62. Ladenson PW, Goldenheim PD, Ridgway EC. Prediction and reversal of blunted ventilatory responsiveness in patients with hypothyroidism. Am J Med 1988;84:877–83.
63. Zwillich CW, Pierson DJ, Hofeldt FD, et al. Ventilatory control in myxedema and hypothyroidism. N Engl J Med 1975;292:662–5.
64. Aagaard C, Christophersen AS, Finnerup S, et al. The prevalence of acromegaly is higher than previously reported: changes over a three-decade period. Clin Endocrinol 2022;97:773–82.
65. Colao A, Ferone D, Marzullo P, et al. Systemic complications of acromegaly: epidemiology, pathogenesis, and management. Endocr Rev 2004;25: 102–52.
66. Davi MV, Dalle Carbonare L, Giustina A, et al. Sleep apnoea syndrome is highly prevalent in acromegaly and only partially reversible after biochemical control of the disease. Eur J Endocrinol 2008;159: 533–40.
67. Vannucci L, Luciani P, Gagliardi E, et al. Assessment of sleep apnea syndrome in treated acromegalic patients and correlation of its severity with clinical and laboratory parameters. J Endocrinol Investig 2013; 36:237–42.
68. Grunstein RR, Ho KY, Berthon-Jones M, et al. Central sleep apnea is associated with increased ventilatory response to carbon dioxide and hypersecretion of growth hormone in patients with acromegaly. Am J Respir Crit Care Med 1994;150: 496–502.

Central Sleep Apnea at High Altitude
From Pathophysiology to Treatment

Elisa Perger, MD, PhD[a,b,*], Sébastien Baillieul, MD, PhD[c]

KEYWORDS

• Central sleep apnea • High altitude • Periodic breathing • Loop gain • Hypobaric hypoxia
• Nocturnal hypoxemia • Chronic mountain sickness. • Sleep quality

KEY POINTS

- High-altitude central sleep apnea (CSA) is characterized by non-rapid eye movement (NREM)-predominant periodic breathing (PB) with central apneas/hypopneas occurring after recent ascent; prevalence and severity increases with altitude.
- Mechanism: altitude-related hypobaric hypoxia → hyperventilation → hypocapnia; when $Paco_2$ falls below the apnea threshold during NREM sleep, central apneas/hypopneas recur, producing PB.
- Acclimatization modulates expression: renal bicarbonate loss alters pH, ventilatory responses increase, and plant–controller interactions evolve over days to weeks.
- Lowlanders versus high-altitude populations (eg, Sherpa) differ in ventilatory control and expression of PB at altitude.
- Descent or supplemental oxygen promptly suppresses CSA; acetazolamide reduces instability via metabolic acidosis. Temazepam and related hypnotics improve sleep continuity in some contexts without worsening oxygenation.

INTRODUCTION

More than 500 million individuals live at altitudes above 1500 m, and over 80 million reside above 2500 m.[1] In addition, an increasing number of people travel or commute to high-altitude regions for occupational, scientific, or recreational purposes. An elevation exceeding 2500 m in the context of rapid ascent is widely accepted as high altitude.[2,3] Exposure to high altitude has direct effects on respiratory physiology. Additionally, disruptions in both sleep architecture and continuity often occur, beginning as early as the initial night. Research on sleep at high altitude has important implications for improving sleep health and quality of life in individuals living in, or traveling to, high-altitude environments.

The effects of high altitude on sleep and breathing are primarily driven by reduced atmospheric pressure, which proportionally decreases oxygen availability and results in a lower partial pressure of inspired oxygen (PiO_2). Interestingly, hypobaric hypoxia has been shown to exert a greater impact on nocturnal breathing and sleep structure than normobaric hypoxia.[4] Regarding sleep, hypobaric hypoxic exposure is associated with reductions in total sleep time, sleep efficiency, slow-wave sleep, and rapid eye movement (REM) sleep, as well as increases in arousal duration and frequency.[5–7] Notably, a substantial proportion of individuals (32%–74%) report poor sleep quality or insomnia at high altitude, particularly during the initial days of exposure.[6,8] Exposure to hypobaric hypoxia also triggers an immediate ventilatory response,

[a] Department of Medicine and Surgery, University of Milano-Bicocca, Milan, Italy; [b] Istituto Auxologico Italiano, IRCCS, Sleep Disorders Center, Milan, Italy; [c] Grenoble Alpes University, HP2 Laboratory, INSERM U1300, Grenoble Alpes University Hospital, Grenoble, France
* Corresponding author. Department of Medicine and Surgery, University of Milano-Bicocca, Milan, Italy.
E-mail address: Elisa.perger@unimib.it

Sleep Med Clin 21 (2026) 343–352
https://doi.org/10.1016/j.jsmc.2026.05.002

Abbreviations	
AMS	acute mountain sickness
ASV	adaptive servo-ventilation
CBF	cerebral blood flow
CMS	chronic mountain sickness
EE	excessive erythrocytosis
HA-CSA	high-altitude central sleep apnea
HCVR	hypercapnic ventilatory response
HVR	hypoxic ventilatory response
NREM	non-rapid eye movement
OSA	obstructive sleep apnea
$Paco_2$	partial pressure in CO_2
PB	periodic breathing
REM	rapid eye movement

followed by gradual physiologic adaptation over days to weeks. These processes specifically alter nocturnal breathing patterns, including the development of apneas and hypopneas, often leading to nocturnal periodic breathing (PB).[5] Historical descriptions of altitude-related PB are commonly attributed to Angelo Mosso, who in 1898 published observations including a tracing from his brother.[9] PB is thought to arise from instability in respiratory control mechanisms caused by hypobaric hypoxia and altered carbon dioxide sensitivity.[7]

In susceptible individuals, and even from first night of exposure to elevations above 2500 m, central sleep apnea related to high-altitude PB (high-altitude central sleep apnea [HA-CSA]) may develop, with increasing prevalence and severity at higher altitudes. At very high altitude (≥5000 m), HA-CSA is common among most sojourners.

HA-CSA typically presents as clusters of 2 to 4 hyperpneas separated by an apnea\hypopnea before the next burst.[10,11] This differs from the crescendo–decrescendo waxing and waning respiratory pattern of Cheyne–Stokes breathing in heart failure and from the irregular, often chaotic central events seen with opioid exposure.[10,12]

Acclimatization, the so-called systemic physiologic and molecular responses to prolonged exposure to high altitude, introduces countervailing forces,[5,13,14] leading to reductions in the prevalence of HA-CSA.[15] Renal bicarbonate excretion gradually offsets the acute hypocapnic alkalosis, permitting ventilation to rise further and Pao_2 to increase. Sympathetic activity and cardiac output are initially elevated, and cerebral blood flow (CBF) is high soon after ascent; over ~2 weeks at ~5000 m, CBF tends to return toward sea-level values despite sustained sympathetic tone.[16] Across this time course, hypoxic and hypercapnic ventilatory responses augment, which can raise loop gain even as Pao_2 improves.[17]

This article integrates the description of HA-CSA mechanisms, clinical expression, ethnic and chronic-exposure perspectives, and management strategies.

PATHOPHYSIOLOGY OF HIGH-ALTITUDE CEREBRAL BLOOD FLOW

Altitude is characterized by hypobaric hypoxia, the severity of which increases proportionally with elevation.[18] Upon arrival at high altitude, hypoxic stimulation of peripheral chemoreceptors in the carotid and aortic bodies increases minute ventilation, a response known as the hypoxic ventilatory response (HVR).[19,20] HVR sensitivity progressively rises over several days of exposure. Contemporary mechanistic models describe respiratory control as a closed-loop negative-feedback system that maintains arterial blood gases within narrow limits, with arterial carbon dioxide tension ($Paco_2$) representing the dominant regulated variable during non-REM (NREM) sleep. At altitude, hypobaric hypoxic-induced hyperventilation lowers $Paco_2$ below the apneic threshold generating a central apnea.[5] Whether isolated apneas evolve into sustained PB depends on the stability of ventilatory control, commonly expressed as *loop gain*.[21–23] Loop gain reflects the product of controller gain (chemosensitivity), plant gain (the efficiency of CO_2/O_2 exchange relative to ventilation), and feedback delay (circulatory and neural latencies). Elevated chemosensitivity combined with delayed and efficient gas-exchange dynamics favors ventilatory oscillations.[22] Thus, for a given ventilatory stimulus, longer subsequent apneas indicate higher loop gain.[22,23] A long-standing view links the severity of HA-CSA to heightened HVR. Additionally, imbalance between hypoxic and hypercapnic chemoreflex gains may independently predispose to PB.[11] Pathophysiology of HA-CSA is summarized in **Fig. 1**.

Maximal ventilatory acclimatization is typically achieved after 4 to 7 days at a constant altitude, coinciding with renal compensation for respiratory alkalosis. HVR is genetically determined, varies widely between individuals and is unaffected by physical training.[3] Classic human studies demonstrate that individuals with greater chemosensitivity develop more pronounced HA-CSA and PB, and that early acclimatization may paradoxically increase PB while improving subjective sleep quality.[16,24] Field observations in trekkers ascending to approximately 5000 m show increasing arousals and central respiratory events during the first days at altitude, followed by partial sleep consolidation despite persistent PB.[16,25] However, it can

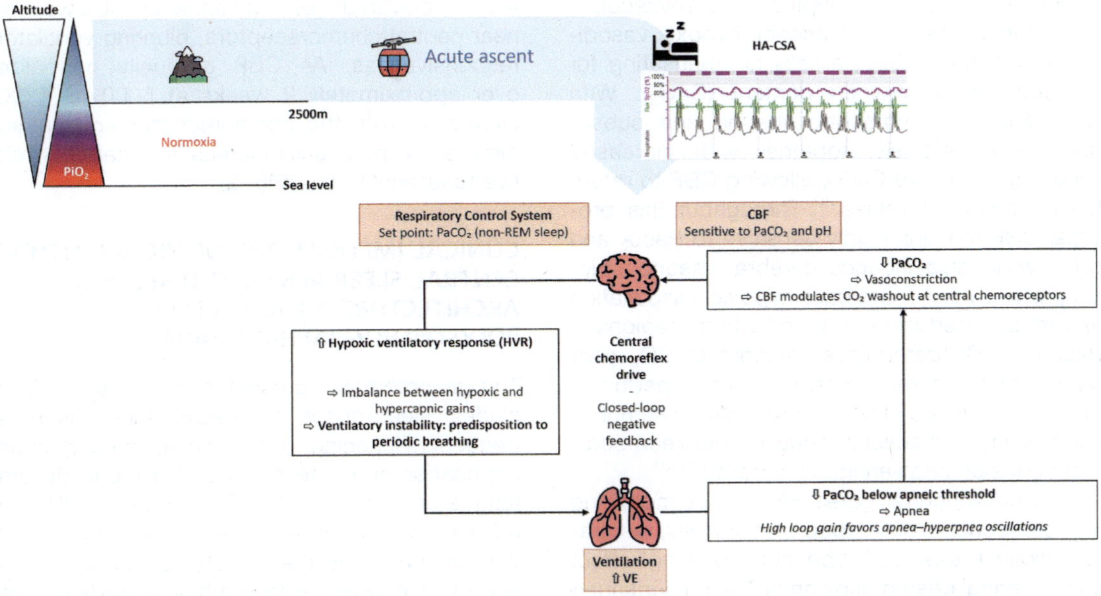

Fig. 1. Pathophysiological mechanisms of acute high-altitude central sleep apnea (HA-CSA): the coupled cerebrovascular–ventilatory model. CBF, cerebral blood flow; HCVR, hypercapnic ventilatory response; HVR, hypoxic ventilatory response; $Paco_2$, partial pressure in CO_2; VE, Minute Ventilation Loop gain = controller gain (chemosensitivity) x plant gain (the efficiency of CO_2/O_2 exchange relative to ventilation) x feedback delay (circulatory and neural latencies).

be modulated by external factors: respiratory depressants (eg, alcohol and sedative-hypnotics) and sleep fragmentation attenuate HVR, whereas respiratory stimulants (eg, progesterone) and sympathomimetics (eg, caffeine and coca) enhance it.[26] As ventilation increases in response to hypoxia, $Paco_2$ decreases and blood pH rises. The resulting alkalosis of the cerebrospinal fluid suppresses central chemoreceptor drive, promoting HA-CSA and attenuating the overall ventilatory response.[27]

Respiratory instability with HA-CSA and PB is most pronounced during NREM sleep, when ventilatory control is dominated by metabolic rather than behavioral mechanisms. At high altitude, sleep architecture is characteristically altered, with a shift toward lighter stages of NREM sleep (stages N1 and N2) and a relative reduction in slow-wave sleep.[6] These architectural changes are not merely epiphenomena but appear to be integrally involved in the pathophysiology of HA-CSA. Light NREM sleep is associated with increased susceptibility to arousals and greater variability in ventilatory drive. Cortical arousals, frequently accompanied by sighs or transient hyperventilation, can acutely lower $Paco_2$. In the context of altitude-induced hypocapnia, such transient reductions are more likely to push $Paco_2$ below the apneic threshold, precipitating CSA. The ensuing apnea promotes CO_2 accumulation, triggering a compensatory hyperventilatory response that may culminate in further arousal, thereby sustaining a self-perpetuating cycle of ventilatory instability and sleep fragmentation.

Moreover, the predominance of lighter NREM sleep reduces the stabilizing influence of deeper sleep stages on respiratory control, further amplifying loop gain and facilitating PB. Rather than being passive markers of disturbed sleep, recurrent arousals play an active role in destabilizing ventilatory control, perpetuating cycles of hyperventilation, apnea, and re-arousal. As a result, sleep instability and arousal propensity emerge as key clinical determinants of altitude-related CSA, linking altered sleep structure directly to the expression and severity of central breathing disturbances.[10,25] Thus, alterations in sleep architecture at altitude both reflect and exacerbate disordered breathing, creating a bidirectional interaction in which sleep fragmentation promotes CSA and PB, while respiratory instability further disrupts sleep structure. This interplay highlights sleep architecture as a fundamental component of the mechanistic framework underlying HA-CSA, rather than a secondary consequence of hypoxia alone.

More recently, cerebrovascular regulation has emerged as an additional contributor to HA-CSA. Larger reductions in CBF at sleep onset are associated with more severe CSA.[28,29] Experimental evidence supports a coupled cerebrovascular–ventilatory model. During ascent, hypoxic vasodilation increases CBF, partially compensating for reduced arterial oxygen content (CaO_2). With acclimatization, hemoconcentration and subsequent erythropoiesis, together with increased ventilation, improve CaO_2, allowing CBF to return toward sea-level values.[30] Throughout this process, CBF remains highly sensitive to $Paco_2$ and pH. Hypocapnia induces cerebral vasoconstriction, which may counteract hypoxic vasodilation and reduce perfusion in specific brain regions.[30] Because CBF determines washout of CO_2 near medullary chemoreceptors, changes in perfusion directly influence the central chemostimulus, establishing bidirectional coupling between cerebral perfusion and ventilatory stability.[30,31]

Acclimatization mitigates HA-CSA by modifying all 3 components of the loop gain. Initially, respiratory alkalosis exerts a "hypocapnic braking" effect on the central chemoreflex drive.[32] With continued exposure, both HVR and the hypercapnic ventilatory response increase, shifting the ventilation–$PaCO_2$ relationship leftward and steepening its slope. This adaptation supports sustained hyperventilation despite alkalosis and preserves chemosensitivity at low $Paco_2$.[30] Progressive bicarbonate excretion restores arterial and brain pH toward neutrality, permitting further increases in ventilation, reductions in $Paco_2$, and improvements in Pao_2 via the alveolar gas equation. Early after ascent, elevated CBF may enhance CO_2 washout near central chemoreceptors, blunting ventilatory responsiveness. As CBF gradually normalizes over approximately 2 weeks at 5000 m,[33] CO_2 clearance from the chemoreceptor environment diminishes, potentially increasing local CO_2 relative to arterial $Paco_2$ (**Fig. 2**).

CLINICAL IMPLICATIONS OF HIGH-ALTITUDE CENTRAL SLEEP APNEA AND SLEEP ARCHITECTURE: INSIGHTS FROM POLYSOMNOGRAPHIC STUDIES

The symptomatic presentation of HA-CSA includes sleep-onset or maintenance insomnia, frequent awakenings (often with air hunger), morning headache, nonrestorative sleep, and daytime fatigue or sleepiness.[6,10] The burden of PB does not always impact sleep quality and fragmentation, underscoring the primary role of hypoxemia and other causes related to high altitude in sleep disruption.[10,11]

Polysomnography or portable monitoring typically reveals central events clustered in NREM with cycle times less than 40 s and event durations of ~10 to 12 s in adults, accompanied by oxygen desaturation of variable depth depending on altitude and physiology.[10] Apnea duration can be shorter than 10 s, which is out of the definition of the respiratory events according to the American Academy of Sleep Medicine (AASM) (at least 10

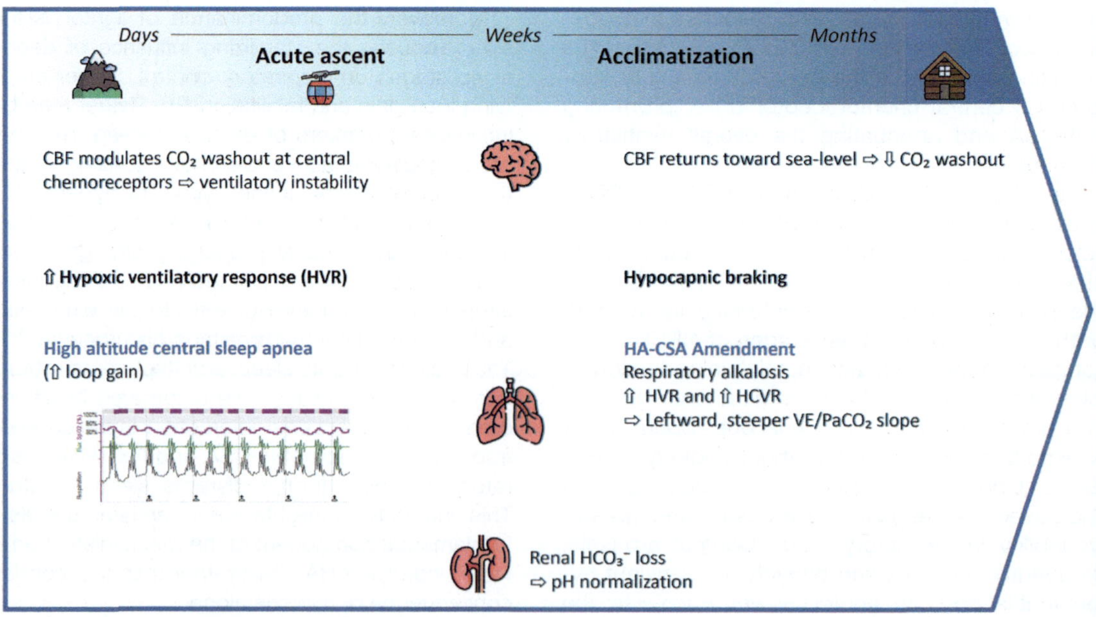

Fig. 2. High altitude CSA: from acute exposure to acclimatization. CBF, cerebral blood flow; HCVR, hypercapnic ventilatory response; HVR, hypoxic ventilatory response; $Paco_2$, partial pressure in CO_2; VE, Minute Ventilation; Loop gain = controller gain (chemosensitivity) x plant gain (the efficiency of CO_2/O_2 exchange relative to ventilation) x feedback delay (circulatory and neural latencies).

s of durations), but adds to the hypoxic and ventilatory burden experienced by subjects at high altitude.[10] **Fig. 3** represent a sample of CSA with PB recorded at HA.

As previously described, at high altitude, HA-CSA and PB occur predominantly during light NREM sleep, where arousals and altitude-induced hypocapnia facilitate $Paco_2$ drops below the apneic threshold. Sleep fragmentation and reduced slow-wave sleep actively destabilize ventilatory control, perpetuating cycles of apnea, hyperventilation, and re-arousal, whereas REM sleep is relatively less affected by cyclic CSA patterns.[6,10]

Coexisting sleep-disordered breathing phenotypes are common. In susceptible subjects with established obstructive sleep apnea (OSA), simulated altitude (eg, normobaric hypoxia at ~15% O_2) can worsen the sleep respiratory disturbance converting the main type of apnea to sustained CSA.[34,35] These effects are explained by hypobaric hypoxia increasing ventilatory controller gain, narrowing the CO_2 reserve, and elevating loop gain, thereby rendering the system more unstable to arousal-related perturbations.[36] Interestingly, altitude exposure in untreated patients with OSA, beyond the increase in sleep-related breathing disturbances due to frequent central apnoeas/hypopnoeas aggravates nocturnal hypoxemia, impairs driving simulator performance and induces cardiovascular stress, including significant increase in mean nocturnal heart rate.[35] These findings highlight the susceptibility of untreated OSA lowlanders to HA-CSA, with implications for counseling and care of OSA patients planning to travel to HA.

Impact of Periodic Breathing on Mean SpO_2

Recent studies converge on the finding that HA-CSA is not responsible for the reduction of mean nocturnal oxygen saturation despite frequent desaturations.[37] When comparing within subjects at a simulated altitude of 3500 m, the average SpO_2 did not differ between periods of regular breathing and PB, if sleep stage and body position were controlled. Additionally, at higher altitudes, increasing HA-CSA severity was not linked to lower mean sleeping SpO_2 across various ascent profiles.[37] Rather, PB increased SpO_2 variability without affecting average oxygenation, consistent with alternating phases of hypoventilation and compensatory hyperventilation that result in a neutral net effect.[38] Importantly, baseline (awake) SpO_2 emerged as the strongest predictor of mean nocturnal SpO_2 in hypoxia, pointing to individual ventilatory acclimatization and chemoresponsiveness as the main drivers of nocturnal oxygenation, rather than CSA burden per se.[37] With ascent, apnea-hypopnea index (AHI)/oxygen desaturation index (ODI) rise and mean/nadir SpO_2 fall as expected, but higher CSA severity does not translate into worse mean nocturnal oxygenation at altitude.[38] This concept provides a physiologic bridge to acute mountain sickness (AMS), the most common form of high-altitude illness, defined as a symptom complex—including headache, nausea, dizziness, fatigue, and sleep

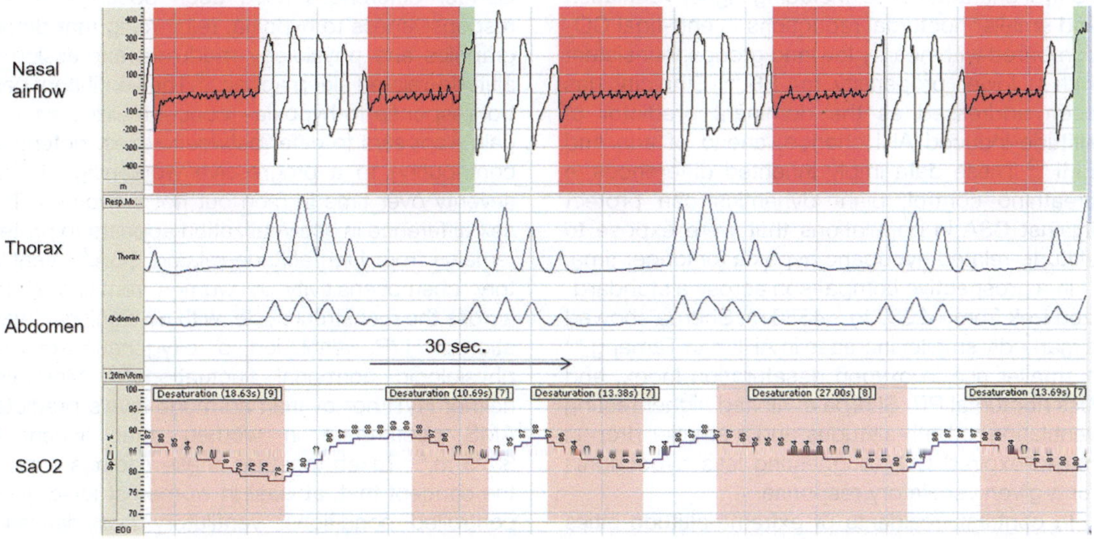

Fig. 3. Sample of CSA (*red squares*) with periodic breathing in a subject living at sea level ascending at 5000 m. First-line represent nasal cannula signal, second and third thorax and abdomen belts, fourth signal oxygen desaturation.

disturbance—that develops within hours to days after ascent and reflects inadequate acclimatization to hypoxia. In this context, the work by Nespoulet and colleagues adds a critical mechanistic layer, showing that individuals susceptible to AMS exhibit reduced peripheral hypoxic chemosensitivity, lower mean nocturnal SpO_2, and fewer central respiratory events during sleep compared with altitude-tolerant subjects.[39] Thus, HA-CSA appears not as a cause of impaired oxygenation, but rather as an epiphenomenon of a high ventilatory drive that may paradoxically preserve mean nocturnal SpO_2 and reduce AMS risk.

Clinically, these data suggest that HA-CSA should not automatically be considered harmful in healthy sojourners or residents, shifting the focus from treating apnoea–hypopnoea indices alone toward identifying individuals with blunted ventilatory responsiveness and clinically relevant symptoms, who may be the ones most likely to benefit from targeted interventions.[38,39] However, the greater SpO_2 oscillations during PB may still have physiologic consequences such as intermittent hypoxia-related oxidative stress and inflammation, sleep fragmentation, and sympathetic activation, warranting context-specific judgment especially in vulnerable populations.[37]

NOVEL PERSPECTIVES

Ethnic Determinants

Population-specific and environmental factors may shape physiologic and pathophysiological responses to HA exposure. High-altitude populations such as Sherpa exhibit distinct ventilatory control characteristics, including higher ventilation and smaller nocturnal reductions in end-tidal CO_2 compared with nearby lowland groups, consistent with a lower propensity for PB.[40] Ethnicity has been addressed as the dominant predictor of altitude-induced AHI change, ahead of age and BMI.[40] These data imply inherited differences in breathing control: plant dynamics can protect against CSA in populations that were expose to altitude-related hypobaric hypoxia for longer time.

In a prospective comparison across a standardized trek from ~2030 to ~4380 m, Sherpa showed a markedly smaller increase in AHI than Tamang,[41] a smaller rise in oxygen desaturation index, and less nocturnal PB. Sherpa exhibited higher resting ventilation at both altitudes and a smaller drop in mixed-expired CO_2, suggesting less hypocapnia for a given ventilatory response.

In contrast, residents of extreme-altitude cities (eg, La Rinconada, ~5100 m) experience profound nocturnal hypoxemia. In these populations, OSA is often the predominant phenotype and may exacerbate altitude-related chronic hypoxemia during sleep. Among individuals with excessive erythrocytosis (EE) or chronic mountain sickness (CMS), mean nocturnal SpO_2 is lower and desaturation nadirs are more pronounced.[42,43] (See also below.)

Extreme Altitude Residency. From Adaptation to Maladaptation

Highlanders are known to develop unique adaptations to chronic hypoxic exposure but also, for some of them, to present a maladaptive syndrome called CMS related to EE and with consequent cardiorespiratory diseases.[44–46] The Expedition 5300 investigations in La Rinconada (~5100–5300 m) document a striking physiology: daytime SpO_2 near ~80%, Pa_{O_2} ~35 mm Hg and Pa_{CO_2} ~34 mm Hg in non-CMS adults, and exceptionally high hemoglobin concentrations and blood viscosity.[47,48] Across lowland Lima (80 m), Puno (~3800 m), and La Rinconada (~5100 m), increasing altitude was associated with lower mean nocturnal SpO_2 (~79% at 5100 m vs ~84% at 3800 m). Within La Rinconada, CMS was associated with lower mean nocturnal SpO_2 (~74% vs ~79% in non-CMS), deeper nadir desaturations (~49% vs ~67%), and higher nocturnal blood pressure variability.[43] These findings link sleep-related hypoxemia with vascular and autonomic stress and EE/CMS progression at extreme altitude.[41,43] In this context, the specific role of CSA beyond hypoxia itself still need to be defined.

Gender Determinants

Gender differences have been observed in PB responsiveness to hypoxia, reinforcing that demographics and physiology modulate expression of altitude-related sleep apnea.[49] The ventilatory control response to hypoxia—conceptualized as loop gain—appears to differ between sexes, potentially contributing to a progressive worsening of CSA severity over time in men but not in women. This sex difference in acclimatization appears to protect females from high altitude-related CSA.[50] Ventilatory chemosensitivity in women remains stable across the menstrual cycle, with no significant variation in HVR, ventilation, or oxygenation despite physiologic hormonal fluctuations.[51] Moreover, neither HVR nor ovarian hormone levels predicted AMS occurrence in women after ascent to 3375 m.[52] Taken together, these findings support the concept that, at least in women studied under controlled conditions, ventilatory acclimatization to hypoxia appears relatively stable across hormonal phases. While sex-related differences in the expression of HA-CSA have been reported, the underlying mechanisms remain incompletely understood and cannot be attributed solely to menstrual hormonal fluctuations. It should also be acknowledged that, similarly to the broader OSA literature—including randomized controlled trials—women remain underrepresented in many studies investigating sleep-disordered breathing. This underrepresentation limits the availability of sex-specific data and makes it difficult to draw definitive conclusions regarding the role of biological sex and hormonal status in the pathophysiology and clinical expression of HA-CSA. Further studies are required to precise the role of biological sex and hormones in HA-CSA pathophysiology.

TREATMENTS OF HIGH-ALTITUDE CENTRAL SLEEP APNEA

Prevalence and severity of HA-CSA increase with elevation. Accordingly, descent is the definitive remedy when feasible. If descent is impractical or temporarily impossible, supplemental oxygen reliably suppresses central events.[53] Correction of hypobaric hypoxemia with supplemental oxygen has been shown to improve sleep apnea at altitude, both in nonacclimatized persons and long-term dwellers.[54,55] However, nocturnal supplemental oxygen may have limitations, particularly as certain circumstances might preclude its use, as it might not be widely available in lowlanders ascending to altitude. In hypobaric environments, achieving normal arterial oxygen tension (Pa_{O_2}) necessitates the administration of higher inspired oxygen fractions (Fi_{O_2}). When oxygen is delivered nasally, local mucosal irritation may occur, and even moderate over-supplementation can exert significant systemic physiologic effects. Moreover, supplemental oxygen may hinder acclimatization by attenuating exposure to hypoxemia. Although a single-night study has shown no alteration in either hypoxic or hypercapnic ventilatory responses, longer-term investigations may be required to fully elucidate potential effects.[56] Some high-altitude working environments, such as mines situated at high altitude, have implemented sleeping rooms enriched by oxygen to help workers adaptations during weekly shifts at high altitude.[57,58] In a randomized, single-blinded, crossover design, 12 men underwent 2 3-day sojourns separated by 4 weeks in hypobaric hypoxia corresponding to 4000 m of altitude, Ibrahim and colleagues tested the impact of increasing inspiratory CO_2 to prevent nocturnal PB.[59] They showed that CO_2 enrichment led to marked stabilization of ventilation during sleep, effectively preventing hypoxia-induced nocturnal PB without affecting sleep macro-architecture, as assessed by polysomnography. Whether this strategy could translate into therapeutic practice require further investigations.

Acetazolamide is effective when administered orally, with multiple studies demonstrating substantial reductions in HA-CSA severity at altitude.[60–63] The predominant mechanism with repeated oral dosing was a mild metabolic acidosis that increases the CO_2 reserve, moving the Pa_{CO_2} level away from the apnea threshold and stabilizing the loop gain,[64] rather than the rapid effect of intravenous infusion of acetazolamide. In fact, acute intravenous acetazolamide exerts minimal immediate effect on acid–base status or ventilatory responses, but increases CBF[28]—likely by preventing CO_2-mediated vasoconstriction in cerebral arteries—and raises Pa_{CO_2} by ~3 mm Hg.[31] These combined actions temporally reduce central events without the delayed metabolic component of oral therapy.

Noninvasive ventilation with bi-level positive airway pressure has also been reported to mitigate high-altitude CSA in selected individuals. However, the underlying mechanism remains unclear, as this approach appears less physiologic for stabilizing ventilatory control. Potential contributors include elevation of mean Pa_{CO_2} above the apnea threshold via intentional rebreathing, altered plant dynamics, and arousal stabilization.[65] Further investigations comparing adaptive servo-ventilation (ASV) with supplemental oxygen demonstrated that ASV was not consistently effective in controlling HA-CSA and PB. Moreover, ASV did not yield significant improvements in oxygenation indices, sleep quality, or related symptoms, apart from a modest increase in mean nocturnal oxygen saturation.[66]

Hypnotic strategies can improve sleep continuity independent of effects on central events. Temazepam and related agents have been associated with better subjective sleep and modest reductions in HA-CSA indices in some studies, with little or no change in average nocturnal SpO_2.[67–69] Nonbenzodiazepine hypnotics have been shown to enhance sleep quality at high altitude without exacerbating oxygen desaturation events.[70] Their use may therefore be considered in selected individuals to improve sleep continuity and restorative rest. However, the administration of any hypnotic agent under hypobaric conditions should be carefully individualized and closely monitored, given the potential variability in physiologic responses and susceptibility to hypoxemia. Additionally, alpinists should be aware of the risk of hypnotics' residual effects in case of an early start for an ascension, with consequences on processing speed and balance control,[71] which may be deleterious for safety and performances of climbers.

In patients with known OSA (treated or not), coexisting HA-CSA management should address both the obstructive and central components of the disorder. Supplemental oxygen or acetazolamide can help suppress central apneas and, in doing so, may reveal residual obstructive events. Once these are unmasked, conventional OSA treatments—such as continuous positive airway pressure can be appropriately titrated to achieve optimal control of both types of events.[72–74]

SUMMARY

HA-CSA is frequent in lowlanders ascending to altitude greater than 2500 m of elevation gain. HA-CSA arises from the convergence of heightened chemosensitivity, sleep-related reductions in respiratory drive, and the gas-, all modulated by cerebrovascular physiology in the presence of hypobaric hypoxia. Acclimatization reshapes these elements over days to weeks, and both clinical manifestations and treatment responses follow from these dynamics. Pragmatic management prioritizes descent or oxygen when necessary. Emerging work linking CBF to ventilatory stability, together with population studies in high-altitude residents, continues to refine this integrated model.

CLINICS CARE POINTS

- Ascent triggers HA-CSA: after rapid ascent above ~2500 m, hypobaric hypoxia can induce hyperventilation, hypocapnia, and NREM-predominant central apneas/periodic breathing.
- Acclimatization reshapes CSA: over days to weeks, bicarbonate loss, rising HVR/HCVR, and changing loop gain can modify CSA severity and expression.
- Descent is definitive treatment: when feasible, descent is the most direct remedy; if not possible, oxygen or drugs may be used to suppress central events.

FUNDING

No funding.

DISCLOSURE

No conflict of interest related to this project.

REFERENCES

1. Tremblay JC, Ainslie PN. Global and country-level estimates of human population at high altitude. Proc Natl Acad Sci U S A 2021;118.
2. Imray C, Booth A, Wright A, et al. Acute altitude illnesses. Br Med J 2011;343:d4943.
3. Merz TM, Pichler Hefti J. Humans at extreme altitudes. BJA Educ 2021;21:455–61.
4. Heinzer R, Saugy JJ, Rupp T, et al. Comparison of sleep disorders between real and simulated 3,450-m altitude. Sleep 2016;39:1517–23.
5. Ainslie PN, Lucas SJ, Burgess KR. Breathing and sleep at high altitude. Respir Physiol Neurobiol 2013;188:233–56.
6. Bloch KE, Buenzli JC, Latshang TD, et al. Sleep at high altitude: guesses and facts. J Appl Physiol 2015;119:1466–80.
7. San T, Polat S, Cingi C, et al. Effects of high altitude on sleep and respiratory system and theirs adaptations. Sci World J 2013;2013:241569.
8. Anderson PJ, Wood-Wentz CM, Bailey KR, et al. Objective versus self-reported sleep quality at high altitude. High Alt Med Biol 2023;24:144–8.
9. Mosso A., Life of man on the high alps. Translated from the 2nd Italian edition by E. Lough Kiesow. T. Fisher Unwin; London, 1898.
10. American Academy of Sleep Medicine. Central sleep apnea due to high altitude periodic breathing: diagnostic criteria and essential features. In: International Classification of Sleep Disorders. 3rd edition, text revision. Darien (IL): American Academy of Sleep Medicine; 2023.
11. Burgess KR, Ainslie PN. Central sleep apnea at high altitude, . Hypoxia Year: 2016. New York: Springer; 2019.
12. Randerath W, Baillieul S, Tamisier R. Central sleep apnoea: not just one phenotype. Eur Respir Rev 2024;33.
13. Mallet RT, Burtscher J, Pialoux V, et al. Molecular mechanisms of high-altitude acclimatization. Int J Mol Sci 2023;24.
14. Smith ZM, Krizay E, Sá RC, et al. Evidence from high-altitude acclimatization for an integrated cerebrovascular and ventilatory hypercapnic response but different responses to hypoxia. J Appl Physiol 2017;123:1477–86.
15. Patrician A, Anholm JD, Ainslie PN. A narrative review of periodic breathing during sleep at high altitude: from acclimatizing lowlanders to adapted highlanders. J Physiol 2024;602:5435–48.
16. Nussbaumer-Ochsner Y, Ursprung J, Siebenmann C, et al. Effect of short-term acclimatization to high altitude on sleep and nocturnal breathing. Sleep 2012;35(3):419–23.
17. Coote JH, Tsang G, Baker A, Stone B. Respiratory changes and structure of sleep in young high-altitude dwellers in the Andes of Peru. Eur J Appl Physiol Occup Physiol 1993;66:249–53.
18. Richalet JP. The invention of hypoxia. J Appl Physiol (1985) 2021;130(5):1573–82.
19. Richalet JP. The invention of hypoxia. J Appl Physiol 2021;130:1573–82.

20. West JB. Physiological effects of chronic hypoxia. N Engl J Med 2017;376:1965–71.
21. Khoo MC, Anholm JD, Ko SW, et al. Dynamics of periodic breathing and arousal during sleep at extreme altitude. Respir Physiol 1996;103:33–43.
22. Javaheri S, Badr MS. Central sleep apnea: pathophysiologic classification. Sleep 2023;46.
23. Burgess KR, Ainslie PN. Central sleep apnea at high altitude. Adv Exp Med Biol 2016;903:275–83.
24. Lahiri S, Maret K, Sherpa MG. Dependence of high altitude sleep apnea on ventilatory sensitivity to hypoxia. Respir Physiol 1983;52(3):281–301.
25. Johnson PL, Edwards N, Burgess KR, Sullivan CE. Sleep architecture changes during a trek from 1400 to 5000 m in the Nepal Himalaya. J Sleep Res 2010;19(1 Pt 2):148–56.
26. Sinclair Avila J, Da Re Gutierrez S, Olivero L, et al. Physiology of high-altitude illness. In: Hidalgo J, Da Re S, D'Almeida AG, editors. High altitude medicine: a case-based approach. Cham, Switzerland: Springer International Publishing; 2023. p. 35–44.
27. Sharma P, Misra K. Chapter 1 - high altitude and hypoxia. In: Misra K, Sharma P, Bhardwaj A, editors. Management of high altitude pathophysiology. London, England: Academic Press; 2018. p. 3–8.
28. Xie A, Skatrud JB, Morgan B, et al. Influence of cerebrovascular function on the hypercapnic ventilatory response in healthy humans. J Physiol 2006; 577:319–29.
29. Savina Y, Pichon AP, Lemaire L, et al. Micro- and macrovascular function in the highest city in the world: a cross sectional study. Lancet Reg Health, Am 2024;38:100887.
30. Hoiland RL, Howe CA, Coombs GB, et al. Ventilatory and cerebrovascular regulation and integration at high altitude. Clin Auton Res 2018;28(4):423–35.
31. Burgess KR, Lucas SJ, Shepherd K, et al. Influence of cerebral blood flow on central sleep apnea at high altitude. Sleep 2014;37(10):1679–87.
32. Moore LG, Huang SY, McCullough RE, et al. Variable inhibition by falling CO2 of hypoxic ventilatory response in humans. J Appl Physiol Respir Environ Exerc Physiol 1984;56:207–10.
33. Lucas SJ, Burgess KR, Thomas KN, et al. Alterations in cerebral blood flow and cerebrovascular reactivity during 14 days at 5050 m. J Physiol 2011;589: 741–53.
34. Burgess KR, Cooper J, Rice A, et al. Effect of simulated altitude during sleep on moderate-severity OSA. Respirology 2006;11:62–9.
35. Nussbaumer-Ochsner Y, Schuepfer N, Ulrich S, et al. Exacerbation of sleep apnoea by frequent central events in patients with the obstructive sleep apnoea syndrome at altitude: a randomised trial. Thorax 2010;65:429–35.
36. Edwards BA, Sands SA, Owens RL, et al. Effects of hyperoxia and hypoxia on the physiological traits responsible for obstructive sleep apnoea. J Physiol 2014;592:4523–35.
37. Heiniger G, Raemy F, Solelhac G, et al. Altitude-induced central sleep apnea does not affect mean sleep oxygen saturation in young healthy males. J Appl Physiol 2025;138:792–8.
38. Bird JD, Kalker A, Rimke AN, et al. Severity of central sleep apnea does not affect sleeping oxygen saturation during ascent to high altitude. J Appl Physiol 2021;131:1432–43.
39. Nespoulet H, Wuyam B, Tamisier R, et al. Altitude illness is related to low hypoxic chemoresponse and low oxygenation during sleep. Eur Respir J 2012;40:673–80.
40. Heiniger G, Walbaum S, Sartori C, et al. Altitude-induced sleep apnea is highly dependent on ethnic background (Sherpa Vs Tamang). High Alt Med Biol 2022;23(2):165–72.
41. Champigneulle B, Brugniaux JV, Stauffer E. Expedition 5300: limits of human adaptations in the highest city in the world. J Physiol 2024;602(21):5449–62.
42. Champigneulle B, Stauffer E, Robach P, et al. Early effects of acetazolamide on hemoglobin mass and plasma volume in chronic mountain sickness at 5100 m. Pulmonology 2025;31(1):2416794.
43. Perger E, Baillieul S, Esteve F, et al. Nocturnal hypoxemia, blood pressure, vascular status and chronic mountain sickness in the highest city in the world. Ann Med 2022;54:1884–93.
44. Monge CM. La enfermedad de los Andes: síndromes eritrémicos. Estudios fisiológicos sobre el hombre de los Andes. Lima, Peru: Imprenta Americana; 1928.
45. Leon-Velarde F, Maggiorini M, Reeves JT, et al. Consensus statement on chronic and subacute high altitude diseases. High Alt Med Biol 2005;6: 147–57.
46. Getu AA, Ilardo M, Tremblay JC, et al. Human adaptation to high-altitude: a contemporary comparison of the oxygen cascade in Andean, Tibetan and Ethiopian highlanders. Exp Physiol 2026;111(3):849–65.
47. Doutreleau S, Ulliel-Roche M, Hancco I, et al. Cardiac remodelling in the highest city in the world: effects of altitude and chronic mountain sickness. Eur J Prev Cardiol 2022;29:2154–62.
48. Champigneulle B, Brugniaux JV, Stauffer E, et al. Expedition 5300: limits of human adaptations in the highest city in the world. J Physiol 2024;602: 5449–62.
49. Lombardi C, Meriggi P, Agostoni P, et al, HIGHCARE Investigators. High-altitude hypoxia and periodic breathing during sleep: gender-related differences. J Sleep Res 2013;22:322–30.
50. Bird JD, Sands SA, Alex RM, et al. Sex-related differences in loop gain during high-altitude sleep-disordered breathing. Ann Am Thorac Soc 2023;20: 1192–200.

51. Citherlet T, Raberin A, Manferdelli G, et al. Menstrual cycle does not impact the hypoxic ventilatory response and acute mountain sickness prediction. Sci Rep 2024;14:26087.
52. Tagliapietra G, Citherlet T, Raberin A, et al. Effect of menstrual cycle phase on physiological responses in healthy women at rest and during submaximal exercise at high altitude. Sci Rep 2024;14:27793.
53. Burgess KR, Johnson PL, Edwards N. Central and obstructive sleep apnoea during ascent to high altitude. Respirology 2004;9:222–9.
54. Luks AM, van Melick H, Batarse RR, et al. Room oxygen enrichment improves sleep and subsequent day-time performance at high altitude. Respir Physiol 1998;113:247–58.
55. Moraga FA, Jiménez D, Richalet JP, et al. Periodic breathing and oxygen supplementation in Chilean miners at high altitude (4200m). Respir Physiol Neurobiol 2014;203:109–15.
56. McElroy MK, Gerard A, Powell FL, et al. Nocturnal O2 enrichment of room air at high altitude increases daytime O2 saturation without changing control of ventilation. High Alt Med Biol 2000;1:197–206.
57. Moraga FA, López I, Morales A, et al. The effect of oxygen enrichment on cardiorespiratory and neuropsychological responses in workers with chronic intermittent exposure to high altitude (ALMA, 5,050 m). Front Physiol 2018;9:187.
58. Perger EC J, Ottolenghi S, Lang M, et al. Intermittent exposure to high-altitude work: nocturnal hypoxemia sea-level anthropometric and biochemical markers. Sleep and Breathing 2026. https://doi.org/10.1007/s11325-026-03751-7.
59. Ibrahim A, Stefani A, Cesari M, et al. Effects of periodic breathing on sleep at high altitude: a randomized, placebo-controlled, crossover study using inspiratory CO(2). J Physiol 2024;602:5549–68.
60. Swenson ER. Respiratory and renal roles of carbonic anhydrase in gas exchange and acid-base regulation. Exs 2000;281–341.
61. Sutton JR, Gray GW, Houston CS, et al. Effects of duration at altitude and acetazolamide on ventilation and oxygenation during sleep. Sleep 1980;3:455–64.
62. Fan JL, Burgess KR, Thomas KN, et al. Effects of acetazolamide on cerebrovascular function and breathing stability at 5050 m. J Physiol 2012;590:1213–25.
63. Fischer R, Lang SM, Leitl M, et al. Theophylline and acetazolamide reduce sleep-disordered breathing at high altitude. Eur Respir J 2004;23:47–52.
64. Schmickl CN, Landry S, Orr JE, et al. Effects of acetazolamide on control of breathing in sleep apnea patients: mechanistic insights using meta-analyses and physiological model simulations. Physiol Rep 2021;9:e15071.
65. Johnson PL, Popa DA, Prisk GK, et al. Non-invasive positive pressure ventilation during sleep at 3800 m: relationship to acute mountain sickness and sleeping oxyhaemoglobin saturation. Respirology 2010;15:277–82.
66. Orr JE, Heinrich EC, Djokic M, et al. Adaptive servo-ventilation as treatment for central sleep apnea due to high-altitude periodic breathing in nonacclimatized healthy individuals. High Alt Med Biol 2018;19:178–84.
67. Dubowitz G. Effect of temazepam on oxygen saturation and sleep quality at high altitude: randomised placebo controlled crossover trial. Br Med J 1998;316:587–9.
68. Nickol AH, Leverment J, Richards P, et al. Temazepam at high altitude reduces periodic breathing without impairing next-day performance: a randomized cross-over double-blind study. J Sleep Res 2006;15(4):445–54.
69. Tanner JB, Tanner SM, Thapa GB, et al. A randomized trial of temazepam versus acetazolamide in high altitude sleep disturbance. High Alt Med Biol 2013;14:234–9.
70. Beaumont M, Batéjat D, Piérard C, et al. Zaleplon and zolpidem objectively alleviate sleep disturbances in mountaineers at a 3,613 meter altitude. Sleep 2007;30:1527–33.
71. Bouzat P, Sechaud G, Banco P, et al. The effect of zolpidem on cognitive function and postural control at high altitude. Sleep 2018;41.
72. Latshang TD, Nussbaumer-Ochsner Y, Henn RM, et al. Effect of acetazolamide and autoCPAP therapy on breathing disturbances among patients with obstructive sleep apnea syndrome who travel to altitude: a randomized controlled trial. JAMA 2012;308:2390–8.
73. Nussbaumer-Ochsner Y, Latshang TD, Ulrich S, et al. Patients with obstructive sleep apnea syndrome benefit from acetazolamide during an altitude sojourn: a randomized, placebo-controlled, double-blind trial. Chest 2012;141:131–8.
74. Schmickl CN, Landry SA, Orr JE, et al. Acetazolamide for OSA and central sleep apnea: a comprehensive systematic review and meta-analysis. Chest 2020;158:2632–45.

Idiopathic Central Sleep Apnea

Sahan Chandrasekara, MBBS, FRACP[a], Matthew T. Naughton, MD FRACP[b,c,*]

KEYWORDS

• Idiopathic central sleep apnoea • Loop gain • Cheyne Stokes respiration

KEY POINTS

- Central sleep apnea (CSA) can be characterized as either *persistent hypoventilation* with hypercapnia (eg, motor neurone disease) or *periodic hyperventilation* followed by a central apnoea associated with normal or reduced CO_2 (eg, opioids, idiopathic, and heart failure).
- Nonhypercapnic CSA, including idiopathic central sleep apnoea (ICSA), occur due to derangements in ventilatory control.
- ICSA describes periodic, nonhypercapnic CSA that occurs in the absence of an identifiable etiology.
- Polysomnographic features in ICSA include short-cycle length central apneas. Arousals have been noted to occur at the termination of the apnoea, rather than the peak of the hyperpnea.
- The natural history of CSA, and consequently the implications of suppressive treatment, is not well-understood.
- We recommend treatment of ICSA focus on identification and reversal of any metabolic/physiologic derangement, monitoring of symptoms and consideration of referral to an expert center.

INTRODUCTION

Central sleep apnea (CSA), a form of sleep disordered breathing, in which there is a failure to drive ventilation. It can be either hypercapnic related to persistent and prolonged hypoventilation or normohypocapnia associated with periodic hyper then hypoventilation with a cycle length (ventilation and apnea periods) usually less than 90 seconds.[1]

Hypercapnic CSA occurs in patients who have persistent and prolonged hypoventilation over days, weeks or years. Etiology of such include primary neuromuscular disorders (eg, motor neurone disease), obesity hypoventilation syndrome, diaphragm palsy or chest wall deformity (eg, kyphoscoliosis). Hypercapnic CSA will not be discussed further in this article.

Periodic nonhypercapnic CSA most commonly occurs in the setting of heart failure, opioid analgesic use, continuous positive airway presure (CPAP) therapy (treatment emergent) or at high altitude in healthy subjects.[2]

Idiopathic central sleep apnea (ICSA) represents a rare subset of CSA patients with no discernible etiologic factor. These patients have a distinct clinical presentation, epidemiology and natural history. The American Academy of Sleep Medicine (AASM) divides CSA into 6 categories (**Box 1**).[3] The biggest group among this is Cheyne-Stokes respiration with CSA (CSR-CSA), the majority of cases of which occur in the setting of cardiac failure.

Specifically, nonhypercapnic CSA is characterized by at least 5 consecutive crescendo–decrescendo patterns of ventilation each followed by a central apnea or hypopnea lasting greater than 10 seconds duration. It is this nonhypercapnic CSA that this article will focus upon.

As will be discussed later, CSA is not a result of upper airway collapse and obstruction as seen with obstructive sleep apnoea.

[a] Alfred Hospital, 55 Commercial Road, Melbourne, 3004, Victoria, Austrlia; [b] Alfred Hospital, Victoria, Australia; [c] Monash University, 99 Commercial Road, Melbourne, 3004, Victoria, Australia
* Corresponding author. Department of Respiratory Medicine, Alfred Hospital, 55 Commercial Road, Melbourne, Victoria 3004, Australia.
E-mail address: m.naughton@alfred.org.au

Sleep Med Clin 21 (2026) 353–364
https://doi.org/10.1016/j.jsmc.2026.06.001
1556-407X/26/

Abbreviations	
AASM	American Academy of Sleep Medicine
ASV	adaptive servoventilation
CSA	central sleep apnea
CSR-CSA	Cheyne-Stokes respiration with CSA
DLCO	diffusing capacity for carbon monoxide
ESS	Epworth Sleepiness Score
FRC	functional residual capacity
GABA	gamma-aminobutyric acid
ICSA	idiopathic central sleep apnea
NIV	noninvasive ventilation
PSG	Polysomnogram
TE-CSA	treatment-emergent CSA
TLC	total lung capacity

EPIDEMIOLOGY

The overall prevalence of nonhypercapnic CSA is significantly higher in men than in women. The reasons for this are not entirely clear. It is plausible that higher average inspiratory muscle strength in men may allow the development of hyperpneas; however, this hypothesis has not yet been tested. It is noted that altitude related periodic breathing occurs to a greater degree, and at a lower altitude, in men compared to women.[4,5]

PATHOPHYSIOLOGY OF NONHYPERCAPNIC CENTRAL SLEEP APNEA

All forms of CSA appear to share a common underlying pathophysiology. This is mediated by 2 primary factors—the apneic threshold and loop gain.

Apnoeic Threshold

In the absence of chronic hypercapnia, ventilation is driven primarily by arterial carbon dioxide levels ($Pa{CO_2}$). In healthy subjects during wakefulness, profound hyperventilation results in hypocapnia and thereby apnea, due to $Pa{CO_2}$ drifting below the *apneic threshold*.[6]

Box 1 American Academy of Sleep Medicine International Classification of Sleep Disorders for Central Sleep Apnoea
Primary CSA
CSA with Cheyne-Stokes breathing (CSR)
CSA due to a medical disorder without CSR
CSA due to high-altitude periodic breathing
CSA due to a medication or substance
Treatment-emergent CSA (TE-CSA)

During rapid eye movement (REM) sleep however, multiple factors beyond a metabolic ($Pa{CO_2}$) drive are responsible for the control of ventilation. This helps explain the irregular rate and tidal volume characteristic of REM sleep.

In contrast, in NREM sleep (especially stage NREM 1 and 2) ventilation is controlled tightly by metabolic drive, most understandably by the prevailing $Pa{CO_2}$ level. As such, the significance of the apneic threshold is magnified in NREM sleep. During normal NREM sleep, $Pa{CO_2}$ increases by up to 3 mm Hg. Normal subjects who are mechanically ventilated demonstrate apneas with modest increases in minute ventilation and reduction of $Pa{CO_2}$ back to waking levels.[7] There also appears to be a more abrupt loss of motor output below the apneic threshold in NREM sleep compared to wakefulness.[8]

These phenomena are mediated by the central and peripheral (carotid body) chemoreceptors. Animal studies suggest that while both central and carotid body chemoreceptor stimulation is required to produce apnea, the effect of hypocapnia on carotid body chemoreceptors is more potent.[9]

Loop Gain

The development of CSA is critically dependent upon a degree of instability in the ventilatory control system. The engineering concept of *loop gain* has been used to describe this, as the ratio of response to a trigger.[9] High loop gain describes a ventilatory system where the degree of ventilatory response is greater than the preceding stimulus related to the period of hypoventilation and relative CO_2 increase, which potentiates cycles of CSA.

There are 3 major components that contribute to loop gain in ventilation (**Fig. 1**).

- Controller gain: ventilatory response to $P{CO_2}$ and a lesser extent $P{O_2}$
- Plant gain: changes in pulmonary capillary blood $P{O_2}$ and $P{CO_2}$ in response to changes in ventilation
- Mixing gain: the delay between gas exchange occurring in the pulmonary circulation and feedback reaching central and peripheral chemoreceptors

Controller Gain

Controller gain describes the responses of the peripheral and central chemoreceptors to $P{CO_2}$/$P{O_2}$. Some circumstances—such as hypoxia or increased sympathetic activity—increase controller gain, that is, changes in $P{CO_2}$ result in greater

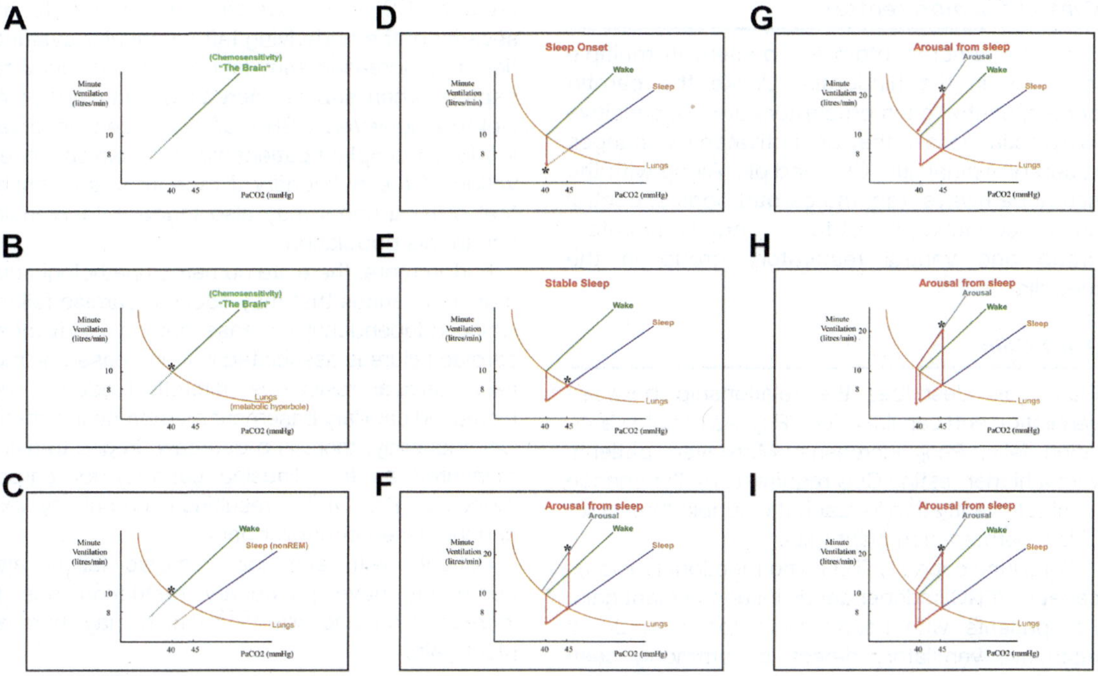

Fig. 1. (*A–I*) illustrates the control of ventilation. (*A*) illustrates the ventilatory response to CO2 (controller gain) and (*B*) overlays the metabolic hyperbole illustrating the effect of ventilation on CO2 (plant gain). (*C*) illustrates the change in chemosensitivity from wake to sleep and the impact upon ventilation (*D, E*). (*F*) illustrates the effect of an arousal on chemosensitivity and increase in minute ventilation, thereby reducing CO2 (*G, H*) followed by a further arousal (*I*).

changes in minute ventilation. Conversely, hyperoxia reduces controller gain—there is a smaller degree of change in minute ventilation in response to changes in P_{CO_2}. An increased controller gain is present in many types of CSA, including ICSA.[9]

The central and peripheral chemoreceptors have complementary roles in modulating ventilatory responses to arterial CO2. Peripheral chemoreceptors, the most significant of which is the carotid body, exhibit a rapid response (10–30 seconds). Central chemoreceptors exhibit a greater magnitude of response, but act more slowly (60–150 seconds)[10(p6)].

The Carotid Bodies

The carotid bodies have a multifaceted and central role in maintaining homeostasis. The functions of the carotid bodies are numerous, with multiple neural pathways, which act in a *ribbon cable* type fashion, that is, the individual pathways may act independently or in tandem. Stimulation of the carotid bodies results in a stimulation of afferent neurons terminating in the nucleus tractus solitarii and resulting in a peripheral chemoreflex.[11]

Most relevant for CSA pathogenesis, the carotid bodies contain multiple chemosensory units that detect changes in P_{CO_2} and arterial pH. Other chemical stimuli include glucose, insulin, hemoglobin and lactate in addition to changes to blood pressure. Following a 10 to 40 second period of hyperventilation, a period of hypoventilation lasting a similar period of time occurs. This hypoventilation results in an increase in P_{CO_2} and decrease in pH, thereby stimulating the carotid body in which causes an increase in respiratory rate and tidal volume.[11]

The carotid bodies also initiate a chemoreflex in response to hypoxia—however, this only begins around a P_{O_2} of 60 mm Hg. In patients with hypoxia and hypercapnia, the additive chemoreflexes produce a large stimulus to ventilation.[10]

Historically, the carotid bodies have been used as a therapeutic target in cardiorespiratory disease, such as severe asthma before the advent of inhaled bronchodilators and inhaled steroids.[12,13] More recently, carotid body resection has been trialed as a therapeutic option to reduce sympathetic drive in heart failure with reduced ejection fraction.[14] Despite meeting the primary endpoint of reducing muscle sympathetic nerve activity, there was significant increase in resting P_{CO_2}.[14]

Central Chemoreceptors

Central chemoreceptors are present in multiple locations in the hindbrain. Unlike the carotid bodies, central chemoreceptors are not sensitive to hypoxia. Rather, they are activated by changes in cerebrospinal fluid CO_2 and pH. Along with the neural pathways from the carotid bodies, central chemoreceptors project to the dorsal respiratory group and ventral respiratory group in the medulla[10(p6),15].

Plant Gain

Plant gain describes the relationship between ventilation and capillary P_{CO_2}/P_{O_2}. As minute ventilation falls, P_{CO_2} increases. Moreover, patients with a higher resting CO_2 require a smaller change in minute ventilation to reach the apneic threshold. This is termed high plant gain.

Total lung capacity (TLC) and functional residual capacity (FRC) independently influence plant gain. For patients with heart failure for example, a restrictive ventilatory defect is commonly seen and is related to cardiomegaly and pleural effusions. For individuals with a lower TLC and FRC, there is a smaller reserve of alveolar O_2 and CO_2 in the lungs. Consequently, a fixed change in minute ventilation will result in a greater degree of change in alveolar and arterial P_{O_2} and P_{CO_2}. This is supported by the observation that there is a decrease in FRC and simultaneous increase in dynamic loop gain in OSA patients during supine sleep, as compared to nonsupine sleep.[16]

CLASSIFICATION OF NONHYPERCAPNIC CENTRAL SLEEP APNEA

Cardiac Failure

Patients with cardiac failure, particularly those with a reduced ejection fraction, generally exhibit a specific type of CSA termed Cheyne-Stokes respiration (CSR-CSA), which is characterized by a long cycle length.[17] Other causes of heart failure exhibit CSR-CSA where cardiac output is reduced due to valvular (eg, aortic stenosis or mitral regurgitation) or rhythm disturbance (eg, atrial fibrillation). A decreased cardiac output leads to an increased arterial circulation time (mixing gain).

Some patients with cardiac failure do not demonstrate normal sleep-related decreases in ventilation and increases in P_{CO_2}, reducing the CO_2 reserve (difference between resting CO_2 and apnoeic threshold).[18]

Some patients with cardiac failure demonstrate awake low Pa_{CO_2} indicative of resting hyperventilation. Despite low Pa_{CO_2} decreasing plant gain, these patients have been noted to have higher rates of CSR-CSA, which is likely due to the severity of the underlying left ventricular dysfunction and increased stimulation of pulmonary J receptors when supine (increased controller gain). Notably however, CSR-CSA has been observed in a lung transplant patient with mechanical denervation of the pulmonary J receptors, suggesting that other triggers may also trigger hyperventilation in this population.[19]

Furthermore, there are numerous pathologic pulmonary changes that may occur in cardiac failure, which independently increase loop gain. Advanced cardiac failure is associated with increased pulmonary vascular resistance, interstitial edema, and increased capillary basement membrane thickness. Consequently, there is a decrease in gas transfer, measured as the diffusing capacity for carbon monoxide (DLCO),[20,21] resulting in chronic hypoxia and increased controller gain.

Patients with advanced cardiac failure also commonly have pulmonary restriction due to increased cardiac size,[22,23] which may increase plant gain.

Opiates

Sleep disordered breathing occurs in approximately 60% of chronic methadone users.[24] Within the sleep disordered breathing (SDB) group, about 20% have CSA and the balance obstructive sleep apnea (OSA). Those with CSA have a lower resting SpO_2 yet maintain or elevate their SpO_2 levels with sleep, compared with OSA and no apnea groups in whom there is a decrease in SpO_2.[25] The relative increase in SpO_2 with sleep is likely due to underlying periodic hyperventilation.

Opiates mediate central sleep apnea primarily through stimulation of mu receptors in the pre-Botzinger complex and parabrachial/Kolliker-Fuse nucleus.[26] Opiate use reduces resting minute ventilation (resulting in a mild increase in Pa_{CO_2}) due to a suppressed central ventilatory response. Of interest is the elevated peripheral ventilatory response with opioids, which results in the periodic hyperventilation followed by apnea characteristic of opioid induced CSA.[27,28] During sleep, this manifests as hypercapnic periodic CSA. However, patients with opiate induced CSA often display an irregular, periodic ventilation pattern termed *ataxic breathing* on PSG.[29] This phenomenon is not seen in other causes of hypercapnic CSA.

CPAP Emergent Central Sleep Apnea

This condition is defined by a residual central AHI of greater than 5 events per hour on CPAP. It occurs in about 5% of patients with significant OSA who initiate CPAP.[30] It self-resolves in the majority of patients within 30 days.

The mechanism responsible may be related to a readjustment of chemosensitivity—chronic intermittent hypoxia and hypercapnia due to OSA are abolished with CPAP, such that triggers for chemosensitivity are changed. An alternative theory relates to excessive CPAP pressures, greater stretch receptor activation via the afferent vagal nerve (Hering-Breurer reflex).[31,32] If there is persistent CSA on CPAP after 30 days despite readjusting pressures, it would be wise to exclude cardiac or opioid related causes. Uncommonly, patients could be trialled on alternative flow generators such as adaptive servoventilation.

In another group, patients with OSA who have been stable on long term CPAP with apnea hypopnea index (AHI) less than 5 events per hour suddenly—over a few days—develop quite a variable residual AHI often between 5 to 30 events per hour. Commonly this is due to the development of atrial fibrillation and carries with it an 14-fold increased risk of a serious cardiac event.[33,34]

Although poorly described in the literature, patients with SDB on auto CPAP who also have periodic limb movements may have a high residual AHI identified from some flow generator devices. It is possible this occurs as a result of the periodic increase in motor activity of intercostal as well as limb skeletal muscles. The transient increase in intercostal activity can change the tidal volume and thereby interfere with the feedback the auto CPAP devices require to set their pressure.

High Altitude

Periodic breathing occurs almost universally at high altitude, even in healthy subjects. As altitude increases Fio_2 decreases, increasing controller gain, and the risk of CO_2 falling less than the apnoeic threshold.[35]

Cerebrovascular Disease

Although obstructive sleep apnea is the most common form of sleep disordered breathing in patients post stroke, a significant number demonstrate CSA. Two distinct patterns have been observed—a CSR-CSA pattern, which occurs in patients with subclinical left ventricular dysfunction[36] and a short cycle length pattern.[9,37] Short cycle length CSA post stroke is likely to be due to changes in ventilatory response to CO_2 (controller gain).[38]

Pulmonary Hypertension

Patients with idiopathic group 1 pulmonary hypertension, by definition, have pulmonary vascular and right ventricular dysfunction but preserved left ventricular function. However, in advanced or decompensated disease there is a diminished cardiac output due to right ventricular failure. This leads to increased mixing gain.[39]

Chronic Renal Failure

Similarly to the cardiac failure population, patients with renal failure are likely to have volume overload and pulmonary edema, which increases controller gain. In keeping with this, the severity of sleep disordered breathing in a population of dialysis patients (including both OSA and CSA) has been shown to improve postfluid removal.[40]

Iatrogenic—Vagal Nerve Stimulators

Vagal nerve stimulation has emerged as a therapeutic option for refractory epilepsy, for which sleep disordered breathing has been reported as a potential complication. Numerous mechanisms have been reported, including in some cases reduction/termination of respiratory effort[41] and hyperventilation with postevent apnea.[42] As the use of vagal nerve stimulators increases, this phenomenon may be observed on a larger scale.

MEDICATIONS

Although opiates are the most commonly implicated medication class, CSA has also been noted with gamma-aminobutyric acid (GABA) receptor agonists and P2Y12 inhibitor ticagrelor.

Gamma-Aminobutyric Acid Agonists

Although less frequently recognized, GABA agonists such as gabapentin, sodium oxybate and valproic acid have been noted to produce CSA with an ataxic breathing pattern. It is likely that the pathophysiology is similar to that of opiate-induced CSA.[43] CSA has also been previously reported in the context of long-term benzodiazepine use.[44]

Ticagrelor

Ticagrelor is an antiplatelet agent that has become widely used in the treatment of acute coronary syndrome. A high prevalence of CSA has been noted in patients taking ticagrelor, which is likely due to an increased hypercapnic ventilatory response.[45,46] Consequently, patients taking ticagrelor may demonstrate polysomnographic findings similar to patients with ICSA. CSA generally normalizes with ticagrelor discontinuation.[46]

The following table outlines the patterns of non-hypercapnic CSA in adults (**Table 1**).

Table 1
Clinical and polysomnographic features of central sleep apnea, grouped by underlying etiology

	Clinical	Cycle Length (sec)	Pa_{CO_2} (mm Hg)	Central Chemoreceptor Sensitivity	Peripheral Chemoreceptor Sensitivity
CSA due to opiates	Positive drug screen	15–45	<50	Reduced	increased
CSA without opiates	Negative drug screen	15–45	<40	Increased	increased
CSA due to heart failure	Low EF, arrhythmia, or valvular disorder	45–75	< 40	Increased	Increased
CSA due to high altitude	Healthy mountain climbers	10–20	<30	Likely increased	Increased
CPAP emergent CSA	Seen with CPAP initiation for OSA	10–20	<40	N/A	N/A

NATURAL HISTORY/PROGNOSIS

As we have outlined, CSA occurs due to a disturbance in normal ventilatory physiology. Unlike OSA, the sequelae of long-term, controlled CSA has not been established. Although CSR-CSA is a negative prognostic marker in cardiac failure, this likely reflects that CSR-CSA becomes more prevalent as severity of cardiac failure increases. For other forms of CSA, its prognostic significance is uncertain.

CSA may in fact be a compensatory mechanism in some contexts. Patients with advanced cardiac failure exhibit resting hyperventilation and increased work of breathing. However, CSR-CSA may improve efficiency of breathing by interspersing hyperpneas with periods of rest (apneas). Further to this, the modest swings in intrathoracic pressure without upper airway obstruction (as with obstructive sleep apnea), which occur during the hyperpnea may improve cardiac output.[47] Also during the periods of hyperventilation, the end expiratory lung volume increases by as much as 1 L. Moreover, the prolonged central apnea is in reality a prolonged exhalation as seen with end tidal P_{CO_2} measurements during CSA. About half way during this *central apnea* the upper airway closes passively, yet pulmonary elastic recoil continues and creates a small amount of PEEP ($\sim$5 cmH_2O), which may be sufficient to prevent alveolar collapse.[47,48]

IDIOPATHIC CENTRAL SLEEP APNEA: A CLINICAL APPROACH

CSA is an uncommon and clinically heterogenous condition. The majority of patients with CSA have an identifiable physiologic etiology, such as cardiac failure, neurologic deficit, or medications. Workup of patients with CSA requires careful evaluation to accurately classify etiology. An estimate of cycle length (from the beginning of hyperventilation to the next is an important guide (**Fig. 2**).

For patients with a reversible physiologic disturbance, treatment should focus on reversal of the specific disturbance where possible. For example, CSR-CSA has been shown to improve with treatment of underlying cardiac failure. These treatments have included pharmacologic,[49] left ventricular assist device,[50] and transplant.[51]

Patients with no discernible etiology and compatible clinical features may have ICSA, for which a uniform management approach has not yet been established. We describe our approach to ICSA here.

Background

ICSA is a rare condition that represents less than 5% of CSA cases.[2,52] ICSA patients present with a unique clinical phenotype, the etiology for which has not yet been described. ICSA patients are more commonly male, and have a median age of between 58.6 and 66.7 in previously described cohorts.[52,53] Although by definition these patients do not have established cardiovascular or cerebrovascular disease, ICSA patients have been shown to have a strikingly high rate of atrial fibrillation,[53] as well as high rates of hyperlipidemia, systemic hypertension[52] and carotid stenosis.[54]

On polysomnography, patients with ICSA demonstrate numerous short cycle length (20–40 second) central apneas, which generally occur in N1 and N2 sleep. Arousals have been observed to occur at the termination of the apnea[2]—in contrast to CSR-CSA, where arousals occur at the peak of ventilation.[55] It has also been noted that the time from sleep onset to stable N3 sleep in increased.[2]

Although the etiology is not completely understood, it has been demonstrated that patients

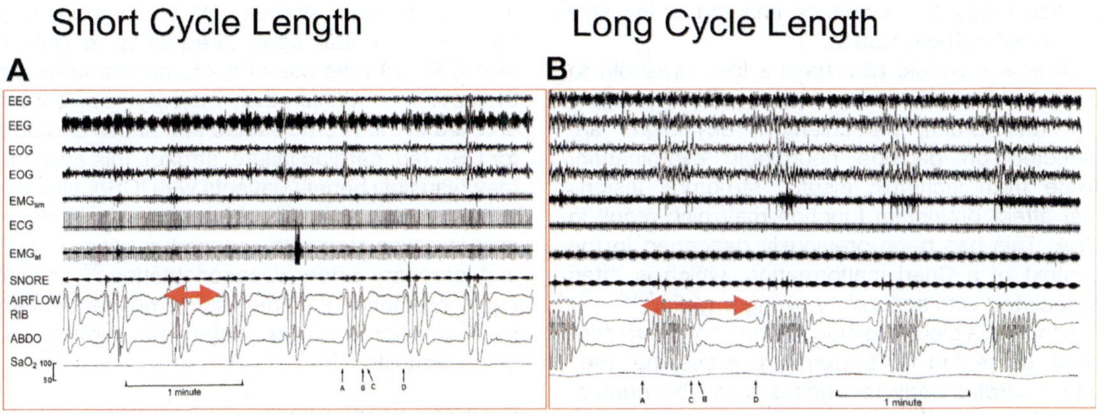

Fig. 2. Two PSGs (4 minute epoch) illustrating the difference between short and long cycle length CSA. Arrows A–B indicate ventilation period and arrows C–D indicate the central apnea. (*A*) represents short CL of 35 seconds: this patient having a normal systolic (LVEF 60%) and diastolic function, in sinus rhythm without valvular heart disease or pulmonary hypertension. In addition absence of diabetes or neurologic impairment. (*B*) illustrates a typical patients with heart failure and CSA-CSR with a long cycle length of 70 sec associated with LVEF 19%.

with ICSA demonstrate increased hypercapnic ventilatory responses, indicative of increased controller gain.[56,57]

Unlike CSR-CSA, which is a negative prognostic marker (in the context of cardiac failure), the prognosis of ICSA are likely relatively benign.[1] However, due to the minority of patients presenting with this condition, further study is required to understand its natural history.

Clinical Presentation

Compared to patients with obstructive sleep apnea, patients with ICSA generally have a lower body mass index (BMI) and are less likely to snore. Both insomnia and hypersomnolence are possible presenting symptoms.[2]

As noted previously, true ICSA is rare. As such, for patients with suspected ICSA we would suggest a robust pathway of investigations to rule out subclinical cardiac or neurologic disease.

Evaluation: a Suggested Approach

A detailed clinical history, including any recent medications, is crucial in patients presenting with suspected ICSA. A urinary drug screen may be considered.

Diagnosis of Central Sleep Apnea

For patients presenting with sleep related symptoms, the initial investigation of choice is an in-lab polysomnogram (PSG). Typically, patients with ICSA will demonstrate sleep state instability, which occurs on the background of multiple central apneas with a short cycle length.

Typically, these patients do not have a high burden of obstructive events. However, note that gold-standard measurement of respiratory effort requires esophageal pressure monitoring, which is seldom performed in routine clinical practice.

Many patients with CSA, including those with ICSA, may demonstrate frequent hypopnoeas on PSG. Identifying central hypopnoeas, as opposed to obstructive, is challenging and not routinely performed by all sleep laboratories. AASM scoring guidelines recommend the use of three metrics to subclassify hypopnoeas, all of which should be absent during a central event.[58]

1. Snoring during the event
2. An increased flattening of the nasal pressure signal compared to baseline
3. Presence of a thoracoabdominal paradox

Supplemental arterial blood gases, which may be accompanied by transcutaneous CO_2 measurements during PSG, may be helpful to demonstrate the presence of hyperventilation rather than hypoventilation.

Exclusion of Identifiable Etiologies

For patients with findings consistent with CSA on PSG, it is then prudent to evaluate for potential underlying etiologies. Given the relatively high prevalence of cardiac failure, particularly among all-comers presenting with CSA, we would suggest measurement of serum naturetic peptides and an initial transthoracic echocardiogram. Patients with subtle abnormalities on these initial investigations may be subsequently referred for cardiac magnetic resonance imaging or invasive right heart catheterization.

Clinicians should also have a low threshold to consider central nervous system (CNS) imaging (eg, MRI brain), particularly if any signs are detected on bedside neurologic examination. Aside from ischemic insults, structural lesions that affect brainstem function may also result in CSA. This has been previously described in the context of a Chari malformation, which is often associated with secondary syringomyelia.[59,60]

Although a clear etiologic link has not been identified, screening for systemic illnesses that may affect carotid body responses could be considered. For example, hyperglycaemia (as may occur in diabetes) and raised serum catecholamines (as may be seen in pheochromocytoma) may impact carotid body signaling.[11]

MANAGEMENT OF IDIOPATHIC CENTRAL SLEEP APNEA

The management of nonhypercapnic CSA, including ICSA, is not well elucidated. Several management options have been trialed, which are detailed further. To date, there have been no large randomized clinical trials of therapy in ICSA. Some management options have been studied more extensively in the CSR-CSA population.

CO_2

Given the fundamental role of hypocapnia in initiating CSA, it has been hypothesized that administration of exogenous CO_2 may increase alveolar CO_2 and subsequently terminate central apnea. This approach has been shown to be effective in reducing AHI, however at the expense of a continuous high respiratory rate and greater arousals in patients with ICSA.[61] In a similar vein, addition of anatomic dead space, which consequently raises arterial CO_2, has been shown to decrease AHI in patients with ICSA.[61]

Despite decreasing AHI, raising arterial CO_2 may independently cause cortical arousals and increase sympathetic tone, which may counteract the improvement in sleep consolidation that occurs with abolition of central apneas.[62] As such, inhaled CO_2 and increasing dead space have not been widely studied, nor have they been adopted as a treatment approaches. In summary, CO_2 therapy is experimental and not used clinically.

Oxygen Therapy

Hyperoxia decreases controller gain, which reduces the magnitude of ventilatory changes relative to changes in arterial CO_2. Several nonrandomized studies have demonstrated decreased central apnea frequency in patients with CSA with the use of nocturnal home oxygen therapy.[63–65] While the majority of patients enrolled in these studies had alternative etiologies for CSA (eg, cardiac failure, stroke), this approach may plausibly benefit patients with ICSA. However supplemental oxygen is not a benign gas. Hyperoxia is associated with reduced cardiac output[66] and coronary artery vasoconstriction.[67] Accordingly, international guidelines do not recommend long term home oxygen therapy for normoxic patients with CHF.[68]

Respiratory Stimulants

Acetazolamide is a carbonic anhydrase inhibitor, which increases renal bicarbonate excretion and results in a mild metabolic acidosis, stimulating respiratory drive. A small nonrandomized study has shown improvement in burden of central apneas as well as clinical symptoms with use of acetazolamide in ICSA patients.[69] Use should be avoided in patients with liver disease or in pregnancy.

Hypnotics

GABAergic hypnotic medications have been trialled in CSA to combat sleep fragmentation. A small trial of 5 patients with ICSA demonstrated that triazolam decreased AHI compared to placebo. However this study was limited by a small sample size, lack of standard deviation measures and lack of quality of life measurements.[70] Two studies have examined the use of zolpidem in CSA (including ICSA), demonstrating a variable reduction in AHI.[71,72] It should also be noted that GABAergic medications, including benzodiazepines, may cause CSA in rare cases.[44]

Continuous Positive Airway Pressure

Continuous positive airway pressure has been shown in select cases to improve central apneas in ICSA.[73,74] It has been postulated that pharyngeal collapse may be implicated in either the initiation and/or propagation of central apneoas, which may account for the therapeutic effect of CPAP.[1] Furthermore, some patients classified as ICSA may in fact have subclinical cardiac disease, and may plausibly have a favorable hemodynamic response from CPAP.

Theoretically, CPAP may increase minute ventilation and therefore increase the chance of P_{CO_2} falling less than the apnoeic threshold, potentiating central apneas—this has been observed in the context of bilevel noninvasive ventilation (NIV).[75] However we are not aware of any documented cases of this in the context of CPAP. Given the potentially heterogenous response to CPAP, in-laboratory titration is suggested to allow retitration to overcome upper airway instability (ie, snoring and obstructive hypopneas) yet avoiding over-zealous over titration.

Noninvasive Ventilation

Typical bilevel fixed pressure NIV is well established as a treatment of disorders of hypoventilation (including hypercapnic CSA) but does not have a role in nonhypercapnic CSA (including ICSA).

Adaptive servoventilation (ASV) is a specific type of bilevel NIV, which has been designed to stabilize breathing pattern in CSA. The ASV algorithm delivers a fixed expiratory pressure, variable pressure support and backup rate.[76] ASV was initially adopted for the management of CSA, particularly CSR-CSA. However, there has been significant controversy regarding its ongoing use in the context of the SERVE-HF trial, which indicated an increased risk of cardiovascular death and all-cause mortality in patients with ASV for patients with heart failure and reduced ejection fraction.[77] This ASV device was triggered by minute ventilation with high pressures.

More recently, the ADVENT-HF trial, which used an alternative ASV algorithm triggered by peak flow with lower pressures, did not reproduce this mortality signal. However, the study may have been underpowered due to the COVID-19 pandemic and Phillips device recall. Another important difference was that the ADVENT-HT trial included a variety of sleep disordered breathing types (obstructive and central).

The use of ASV for CSA is highly variable. The European Respiratory Society and European Sleep Research Society recently published a statement promoting the use of ASV, including in patients with an left ventricular ejection fraction (LVEF) between 30% and 45% (but only when initiation is performed in an expert center).[78]

Phrenic Nerve Stimulation

Phrenic nerve stimulation is a novel and emerging therapy for CSA, including ICSA. Akin to cardiac pacing, phrenic nerve stimulation uses a generator and transvenous lead to stimulate unilateral diaphragmatic contraction. The largest studies of phrenic nerve stimulation in CSA are the pivotal study and follow-up postapproval study, which enrolled patients with CSA of any cause except opiates. 11% of initial patients had idiopathic CSA. Phrenic nerve stimulation was highly effective in reducing AHI and reducing Epworth Sleepiness Score (ESS).[79] However, it should be noted that baseline ESS was in the *high normal* rather than *abnormal range*, likely reflecting the fact that CSA patients often present with insomnia rather than pathologic sleepiness.

Despite significant improvement in AHI and reduction index, patients demonstrated persistently minimal proportions of N3 sleep at 5 year follow-up (1% of total sleep time, compared to 2% at baseline). This may suggest that phrenic nerve stimulation independently influences sleep architecture. Furthermore, there was no monitoring of respiratory symptoms or lung function.

MANAGEMENT: OUR SUGGESTED APPROACH

ICSA is an uncommon condition. Although respiratory effort is routinely quantified during PSG using thoracic and abdominal movement, studies with esophageal manometry demonstrate that respiratory events are often misclassified. Further to this, some patients with true ICSA appear to respond to CPAP, which plausibly may play a role in reversing the underlying physiologic derangement (as in CSR-CSA). As such, we would suggest an initial trial of CPAP for all patients with a suspected diagnosis of ICSA, preferably with an in-lab CPAP implementation study.

For patients who do not respond to CPAP, we would suggest referral to a specialist center for consideration of further management. Quite often in the absence of snoring or any underlying cause (as listed earlier)—observation may be all that is required. Feasible options that may be trialed in this setting with close monitoring include low flow oxygen, acetazolamide, ASV and phrenic nerve stimulation.

In the setting of ICSA, we would suggest reserving phrenic nerve stimulation for carefully selected patients.

FUTURE DIRECTIONS

The clinical entity of ICSA is likely to evolve significantly in the future. Although there is currently no clearly defined etiology, the epidemiologic profile of ICSA suggests that this may be a largely acquired, rather than genetic illness. There may also be heterogeneity within this patient group, which has not yet been described.

Patients with ICSA have high rates of metabolic and cardiovascular comorbidities. As our diagnostic tools improve—or example, use of cardiac MRI (cMRI) over echocardiography in appropriate cases—it is likely that our understanding and classification of this condition will change.

Both current therapeutic options and our understanding of the underlying pathogenesis in ICSA are relatively rudimentary. CSA syndromes may in part reflect an adaptive response to physiologic dysregulation, and the natural history of untreated CSA is not well understood in any context. As our understanding of this condition evolves, evaluation of potential therapies on a broader scale is also warranted. Given that we do not understand the prognostic implications of suppressing CSA, treatments should improve quality of life in addition to reducing the burden of respiratory events.

SUMMARY

ICSA is a rare condition characterized by short-cycle central apneas, which usually occur in transitional sleep. ICSA occurs in the absence of known cardiac failure or established cerebrovascular disease. Data on therapeutic options for ICSA remain relatively sparse; however, there has been significant interest recently in ASV and phrenic nerve stimulation. An evolving understanding of this condition and therapeutic options will serve to improve care for ICSA patients in the future.

CLINICS CARE POINTS

- When CSA appears consider the cycle length: short (<45 seconds indicates opioid induced; long (>45 seconds) indicates heart failure related.
- The pathogenesis of CSA differs significantly from OSA and may not carry the same adverse pathophysiological consequences.
- Evidence suggests treatment of CSA is best directed at the cause (eg opioids, heart failure) rather than the downstream AHI.

DISCLOSURE

None.

REFERENCES

1. Bradley TD, Phillipson EA. Central sleep apnea. Clin Chest Med 1992;13(3):493–505.
2. Eckert DJ, Jordan AS, Merchia P, et al. Central sleep apnea. Chest 2007;131(2):595–607.
3. International classification of sleep disorders—Third Edition (ICSD-3). 3rd edition. Darien (IL): American Academy of Sleep Medicine; 2014.
4. Lombardi C, Meriggi P, Agostoni P, et al. High-altitude hypoxia and periodic breathing during sleep: gender-related differences. J Sleep Res 2013;22(3):322–30.
5. Pramsohler S, Schilz R, Patzak A, et al. Periodic breathing in healthy young adults in normobaric hypoxia equivalent to 3500 m, 4500 m, and 5500 m altitude. Sleep Breath 2019;23(2):703–9.
6. Meah MS, Gardner WN. Post-hyperventilation apnoea in conscious humans. J Physiol 1994;477(3):527–38.
7. Henke KG, Arias A, Skatruo JB, et al. Inhibition of inspiratory muscle activity during sleep: Chemical and nonchemical influences. Am Rev Respir Dis 1988;138(1):8–15.
8. Leevers AM, Simon PM, Dempsey JA. Apnea after normocapnic mechanical ventilation during NREM sleep. J Appl Physiol 1994;77(5):2079–85.
9. Javaheri S, Dempsey JA. Central sleep apnea. Compr Physiol 2013;3(1):141–63.
10. Vassilakopoulos T. Chapter 6 - control of ventilation and respiratory muscles. In: Spiro SG, Silvestri GA, Agustí A, editors. Clinical respiratory medicine. 4th Edition. Amsterdam, Netherlands: W.B. Saunders; 2012. p. 50–62. https://doi.org/10.1016/B978-1-4557-0792-8.00006-4.
11. Zera T, Moraes DJA, Da Silva MP, et al. The logic of carotid body connectivity to the brain. Physiology 2019;34(4):264–82.
12. Nakayama K. Surgical removal of the carotid body for bronchial asthma. Aust N Z J Surg 1962;31(3):214–21.
13. Stulbarg MS, Winn WR, Kellett LE. Bilateral carotid body resection for the relief of dyspnea in severe chronic obstructive pulmonary disease: Physiologic and clinical observations in three patients. Chest 1989;95(5):1123–8.
14. Niewinski P, Janczak D, Rucinski A, et al. Carotid body resection for sympathetic modulation in systolic heart failure: results from first-in-man study. Eur J Heart Fail 2017;19(3):391–400.
15. Nattie E, Li A. Central chemoreceptors: locations and functions. Compr Physiol 2012;2(1):221–54.
16. Joosten SA, Landry SA, Sands SA, et al. Dynamic loop gain increases upon adopting the supine body position during sleep in patients with obstructive sleep apnoea. Respirology 2017;22(8):1662–9.
17. Solin P, Roebuck T, Swieca J, et al. Effects of cardiac dysfunction on non-hypercapnic central sleep apnea. Chest 1998;113(1):104–10.
18. Xie A, Skatrud JB, Puleo DS, et al. Apnea–hypopnea threshold for CO_2 in patients with congestive heart failure. Am J Respir Crit Care Med 2002;165(9):1245–50.
19. Solin P, Snell G, Williams T, et al. Central sleep apnoea in congestive heart failure despite vagal denervation after bilateral lung transplantation. Eur Respir J 1998;12(2):495–8.
20. Kee K, Naughton MT. Heart failure and the lung. Circ J 2010;74(12):2507–16.

21. Szollosi I, Thompson BR, Krum H, et al. Impaired pulmonary diffusing capacity and hypoxia in heart failure correlates with central sleep apnea severity. Chest 2008;134(1):67–72.
22. Olson TP, Beck KC, Johnson JB, et al. Competition for intrathoracic space reduces lung capacity in patients with chronic heart failure. Chest 2006;130(1):164–71.
23. Wright RS, Levine MS, Bellamy PE, et al. Ventilatory and diffusion abnormalities in potential heart transplant recipients. Chest 1990;98(4):816–20.
24. Chung F, Wong J, Bellingham G, et al. Predictive factors for sleep apnoea in patients on opioids for chronic pain. BMJ Open Respir Res 2019;6(1):e000523.
25. Wang D, Yee B, Wu J, et al. Opioid-related central sleep apnea doesn't harm respiratory and sleep parameters. Sleep Adv 2025;6(Suppl 1):A22.
26. Bachmutsky I, Wei XP, Kish E, et al. Opioids depress breathing through two small brainstem sites. eLife 2020;9:e52694.
27. Weil JV, McCullough RE, Kline JS, et al. Diminished ventilatory response to hypoxia and hypercapnia after morphine in normal man. N Engl J Med 1975;292(21):1103–6.
28. Teichtahl H, Wang D, Cunnington D, et al. Ventilatory responses to hypoxia and hypercapnia in stable methadone maintenance treatment patients. Chest 2005;128(3):1339–47.
29. Correa D, Farney RJ, Chung F, et al. Chronic opioid use and central sleep apnea: a review of the prevalence, mechanisms, and perioperative considerations. Anesth Analg 2015;120(6):1273–85.
30. Mador MJ. Emergent central sleep apnea during CPAP therapy-clinical implications. J Thorac Dis 2017;9(11):4182–4.
31. Noah WH, Messineo L, Hete B, et al. Treatment-emergent central sleep apnea resolves with lower inspiratory pressure. J Clin Sleep Med 2025;21(3):559–64.
32. Lombardi C, Caravita S, Parati G. Central sleep apnea during continuous positive airway pressure therapy in obstructive sleep apnea patients: from the compliance to adaptation, maladaptation and reflexes. J Thorac Dis 2017;9(11):4152–6.
33. Naughton MT. The importance of being apnoeic (on CPAP). Respirology 2022;27(2):105–6.
34. Prigent A, Pellen C, Texereau J, et al. CPAP telemonitoring can track cheyne–stokes respiration and detect serious cardiac events: the AlertApnée study. Respirology 2022;27(2):161–9.
35. White DP, Gleeson K, Pickett CK, et al. Altitude acclimatization: influence on periodic breathing and chemoresponsiveness during sleep. J Appl Physiol 1987;63(1):401–12.
36. Nopmaneejumruslers C, Kaneko Y, Hajek V, et al. Cheyne-stokes respiration in stroke: relationship to hypocapnia and occult cardiac dysfunction. Am J Respir Crit Care Med 2005;171(9):1048–52.
37. Parra O, Arboix A, Bechich S, et al. Time course of sleep-related breathing disorders in first-ever stroke or transient ischemic attack. Am J Respir Crit Care Med 2000;161(2):375–80.
38. Baillieul S, Bailly S, Detante O, et al. Sleep-disordered breathing and ventilatory chemosensitivity in first ischaemic stroke patients: a prospective cohort study. Thorax 2022;77(10):1006–14.
39. Schulz R, Baseler G, Ghofrani HA, et al. Nocturnal periodic breathing in primary pulmonary hypertension. Eur Respir J 2002;19(4):658–63.
40. Lyons OD, Chan CT, Yadollahi A, et al. Effect of ultrafiltration on sleep apnea and sleep structure in patients with end-stage renal disease. Am J Respir Crit Care Med 2015;191(11):1287–94.
41. Papacostas SS, Myrianthopoulou P, Dietis A, et al. Induction of central-type sleep apnea by vagus nerve stimulation. Electromyogr Clin Neurophysiol 2007;47(1):61–3.
42. Forde I, Mansukhani M, Kolla B, et al. A potential novel mechanism for vagus nerve stimulator-related central sleep apnea. Children 2017;4(10):86.
43. Javaheri S, Randerath WJ, Safwan Badr M, et al. Medication-induced central sleep apnea: a unifying concept. Sleep 2024;47(8):zsae038.
44. Chakrabarti S, Darisetty S, Gupta N, et al. Masking of obstructive sleep apnoea by drug induced central sleep apnoea. Adv Respir Med 2019;87(3):189–93.
45. Revol B, Jullian-Desayes I, Tamisier R, et al. Ticagrelor and central sleep apnea. J Am Coll Cardiol 2018;71(20):2378–9.
46. Giannoni A, Emdin M, Passino C. Cheyne–stokes respiration, chemoreflex, and ticagrelor-related dyspnea. N Engl J Med 2016;375(10):1004–6.
47. Naughton MT. PRO: persistent central sleep apnea/hunter-cheyne-stokes breathing, despite best guideline-based therapy of heart failure with reduced ejection fraction, is a compensatory mechanism and should not be suppressed. J Clin Sleep Med 2018;14(06):909–14.
48. Naughton MT. Cheyne–stokes respiration: friend or foe? Thorax 2012;67(4):357.
49. Solin P, Bergin P, Richardson M, et al. Influence of pulmonary capillary wedge pressure on central apnea in heart failure. Circulation 1999;99(12):1574–9.
50. Harun NS, Leet A, Naughton MT. Improvement in sleep-disordered breathing after insertion of left ventricular assist device. Ann Am Thorac Soc 2013;10(3):272–3.
51. Mansfield DR, Solin P, Roebuck T, et al. The effect of successful heart transplant treatment of heart failure on central sleep apnea. Chest 2003;124(5):1675–81.
52. Kouri I, Kolla BP, Morgenthaler TI, et al. Frequency and outcomes of primary central sleep apnea in

a population-based study. Sleep Med 2020;68: 177–83.

53. Leung RST, Huber MA, Rogge T, et al. Association between atrial fibrillation and central. Sleep Apnea 2005;28(12):1543–6.
54. Rupprecht S, Hoyer D, Hagemann G, et al. Central sleep apnea indicates autonomic dysfunction in asymptomatic carotid stenosis: a potential marker of cerebrovascular and cardiovascular risk. Sleep 2010;33(3):327–33.
55. Trinder J, Merson R, Rosenberg JI, et al. Pathophysiological interactions of ventilation, arousals, and blood pressure oscillations during cheyne–stokes respiration in patients with heart failure. Am J Respir Crit Care Med 2000;162(3):808–13.
56. Solin P, Roebuck T, Johns DP, et al. Peripheral and central ventilatory responses in central sleep apnea with and without congestive heart failure. Am J Respir Crit Care Med 2000;162(6):2194–200.
57. Xie A, Rutherford R, Rankin F, et al. Hypocapnia and increased ventilatory responsiveness in patients with idiopathic central sleep apnea. Am J Respir Crit Care Med 1995;152(6):1950–5.
58. Troester MM, Quan SF, Berry RB, et al. The AASM manual for the scoring of sleep and associated events: rules, terminology and technical specifications. Darien (IL): American Academy of Sleep Medicine; 2023.
59. Abenza Abildúa MJ, Gutiérrez VL, García JG, et al. Central apnea-hypopnea syndrome and Chiari malformation type 1: pre and post-surgical studies. Sleep Med 2021;88:25–8.
60. Gagnadoux F, Meslier N, Svab I, et al. Sleep-disordered breathing in patients with Chiari malformation: improvement after surgery. Neurology 2006;66(1): 136–8.
61. Xie A, Rankin F, Rutherford R, et al. Effects of inhaled CO_2 and added dead space on idiopathic central sleep apnea. J Appl Physiol 1997;82(3):918–26.
62. Szollosi I, Jones M, Morrell MJ, et al. Effect of CO2 inhalation on central sleep apnea and arousals from sleep. Respiration 2004;71(5):493–8.
63. Franklin KA, Sahlin C, Lundgren R, et al. Reversal of central sleep apnea with oxygen. Chest 1997; 111(1):163–9.
64. Javaheri S, Ahmed M, Parker TJ, et al. Effects of nasal O2 on sleep-related disordered breathing in ambulatory patients with stable heart failure. Sleep 1999;22(8):1101–6.
65. Hanly PJ, Millar TW, Steljes DG, et al. The effect of oxygen on respiration and sleep in patients with congestive heart failure. Ann Intern Med 1989;111-(10):777–82.
66. Haque WA, Boehmer J, Clemson BS, et al. Hemodynamic effects of supplemental oxygen administration in congestive heart failure. J Am Coll Cardiol 1996;27(2):353–7.
67. Guensch DP, Fischer K, Yamaji K, et al. Effect of hyperoxia on myocardial oxygenation and function in patients with stable multivessel coronary artery disease. J Am Heart Assoc 2020;9(5):e014739.
68. Clark AL, Johnson M, Fairhurst C, et al. Does home oxygen therapy (HOT) in addition to standard care reduce disease severity and improve symptoms in people with chronic heart failure? A randomised trial of home oxygen therapy for patients with chronic heart failure. Health Technol Assess 2015;19(75): 1–120.
69. White DP, Zwillich CW, Pickett CK, et al. Central sleep apnea: improvement with acetazolamide therapy. Arch Intern Med 1982;142(10):1816–9.
70. Bonnet MH, Dexter JR, Arand DL. The effect of triazolam on arousal and respiration in central sleep apnea patients. Sleep 1990;13(1):31–41.
71. Quadri S, Drake C, Hudgel DW. Improvement of idiopathic central sleep apnea with zolpidem. J Clin Sleep Med 2009;05(02):122–9.
72. Ahmad B, Sankari A, Eshraghi M, et al. Effect of Zolpidem on nocturnal arousals and susceptibility to central sleep apnea. Sleep Breath 2023;27(1): 173–80.
73. Hoffstein V, Slutsky AS. Central sleep apnea reversed by continuous positive airway pressure. Am Rev Respir Dis 1987;135(5):1210–2.
74. Issa FG, Sullivan CE. Reversal of central sleep apnea using nasal CPAP. Chest 1986;90(2):165–71.
75. Johnson KG, Johnson DC. Bilevel positive airway pressure worsens central apneas during sleep. Chest 2005;128(4):2141–50.
76. Javaheri S, Brown LK, Randerath WJ. Positive airway pressure therapy with adaptive servoventilation. Chest 2014;146(2):514–23.
77. Cowie MR, Woehrle H, Wegscheider K, et al. Adaptive servo-ventilation for central sleep apnea in systolic heart failure. N Engl J Med 2015;373(12): 1095–105.
78. Randerath WJ, Schiza SE, Arzt M, et al. European Respiratory Society and European Sleep Research Society statement on the treatment of central sleep apnoea with adaptive servo-ventilation. Eur Respir J 2025;66(2):2500263.
79. Costanzo MR, Javaheri S, Ponikowski P, et al. Transvenous phrenic nerve stimulation for treatment of central sleep apnea: five-year safety and efficacy outcomes. Nat Sci Sleep 2021;13:515–26.

Central Apnoea in Infants
Apnoea of Prematurity and Apnoea of Infancy

Maysaa Banjari, MD[a,b], Juliann M. Di Fiore, BS[c], Maria Casalino, MD[d], Estelle B. Gauda, MD[e,f,g,h,*]

KEYWORDS

• Loop-gain • Apnea of prematurity • Apnea of infancy

KEY POINTS

- Gestational age, postnatal age and whether apnea is new or increasing in frequency distinguish normal maturational physiology or pathological apnea.
- Immature respiratory control and increased loop gain predisposes premature infants to central apnea, post-sign apnea and periodic breathing; CPAP and caffiene lower loop gain.
- Term infants with persistent or severe central apnea should be evaluated for neurological, metabolic and genetic disorders including congenital central hypoventilation syndrome.
- Central apnea may be the only clinical sign of seizures and should be assessed with continuous video EEG.
- Term or premature infants with new onset or increased frequency or severity of apnea should be evaluated for bacterial or viral infection.

INTRODUCTION

Infants born premature and those born at term can have unstable breathing with recurrent episodes of central apnea requiring intervention for adequate ventilation and oxygenation. In this article, we present the pathophysiology and treatment of apnea in preterm infants using the construct of loop-gain. We also present and discuss the diagnostic criteria, pathophysiology, assessment and treatment of central apnea of infancy, and the importance of polysomnography as key part of the diagnostic workup its use to assess the efficacy of therapeutic interventions.

Apnea of Prematurity: Expression of an Immature Respiratory Network

Apnea of Prematurity (AoP) is defined by the American Academy of Pediatrics as the "cessation of breathing for 20 seconds or longer, or a shorter pause accompanied by bradycardia (<100 beats per minute), cyanosis, or pallor" in neonates born before 37 weeks' gestation. The frequency of apnea is inversely related to gestational age and is essentially universal in infants born $\leq$ 30 weeks gestation. Apnea and intermittent hypoxemia (IH) emerge within a few days after birth, peak by 3 to 4 weeks, then begin to resolve by 10 to 12 weeks

[a] Division of Neonatology, The Hospital for Sick Children, University of Toronto, Toronto, ON, Canada; [b] Department of Pediatrics, King Abdulaziz University, Jeddah, Saudi Arabia; [c] Division of Neonatology, Department of Pediatrics, Rainbow Babies & Children's Hospital, Case Western Reserve University, Cleveland, OH, USA; [d] Department of Pediatrics, Queen's University, Kingston, ON, Canada; [e] Department of Pediatrics, University of Toronto; [f] Division of Neonatology, University of Toronto; [g] Translational Medicine Program, SickKids Research Institute; [h] Toronto Centre for Neonatal Health, The Patient Support Center, The Hospital for Sick Children, Toronto, ON, Canada
* Corresponding author. University of Toronto, The Hospital for Sick Children, The Patient Support Center, 175 Elizabeth Street, Toronto, ON M5G 2G3, Canada.
E-mail address: estelle.gauda@sickkids.ca

Sleep Med Clin 21 (2026) 365–376
https://doi.org/10.1016/j.jsmc.2026.06.002

Abbreviations	
AASM	American Academy of Sleep Medicine
AoP	apnea of prematurity
BRUE	brief resolved unexplained event
CAI	central apnea index
CAP	caffeine for apnea of prematurity
CCHS	congenital central hypoventilation syndrome
CPAP	continuous positive airway pressure
FRC	functional residual capacity
GER	gastroesophageal reflux
IH	intermittent hypoxemia
IL-1β	interleukin-1β
pF	parafacial
PGE_2	prostaglandin E_2
PMA	post-menstrual age
preBötC	pre-Bötzinger complex
RTN	retrotrapezoid nucleus
SIDS	sudden infant death syndrome

postnatal age.[1] However, some extremely preterm infants may still have cardiorespiratory events that prolong hospitalization beyond term gestation.[2] Periodic breathing is defined as at least 3 cycles of alternating respiration and respiratory pauses, occur more often in infants greater than 30 weeks gestation age, emerges 1 to 2 weeks after birth, peaks at 34 to 36 weeks post-menstrual age (PMA),[1,3] then declines and resolves within 6 months post-term.[4]

In the narrow upper airway of the premature infant, the pharynx is the most compliant segment and most common site of obstruction, especially during head flexion.[5] Upper airway muscle activation often occurs slightly before that of the diaphragm to maintain upper airway.[6] However, pre-activation of upper airway muscles in premature infants does not always occur.[7] Thus, vast majority of apnea are central or mixed in nature indicating a reduced level of central respiratory drive.[8]

The pathophysiology of IH differs from that of central apneas. Apneas lasting for 5 to 20 seconds, at adequate functional residual capacity (FRC), even in premature infants with small lung volumes should not cause rapid hemoglobin desaturation. We propose that the convergence of hypersensitivity of arterial chemoreceptor and reduction in FRC in premature infants with evolving lung disease creates the perfect storm for IH to slowly emerge after delivery, and peaking at 3 to 4 weeks PMA.[9] The stage of sleep influences the level of FRC and the frequency of IH. As depicted in **Fig. 1**, premature infants sleep 90% of the time and they are in active, rapid eye movement (REM)-like sleep for 70% to 80% of total sleep time.[10] Apneas are more frequent in active sleep.[11,12] During active sleep, the infant has rapid eye movements, sporadic limb and body movements, myoclonus, and tonic inhibition of upper airway and intercostal muscles, increasing the propensity for upper airway collapse.[13] Moreover, postinspiratory activity of the diaphragm (diaphragmatic breaking) and reduced expiratory activity of the thyroarytenoid muscle, responsible for laryngeal breaking, are inhibited; both function to retard expiration and retain FRC. Low lung volumes precipitate rapid decreases in Hgb saturation.[14] With maturation, the proportion of quiet, (non-REM) to active sleep increases. In quiet sleep, breathing is primarily driven by the level of $Paco_2$. Concurrently, with maturation Pco_2 chemosensitivity is increasing, activity from peripheral arterial chemoreceptors is better integrated within the network such that by 34 to 36 weeks PMA apneas and IH are resolving. IH and apneas beyond 36 weeks PMA, may persist in infants born at less than 26 weeks, especially those with lung disease.[2] A recent study found that in a cohort of premature infants, during wakefulness at 32-week and 36-week PMA, IH was more often associated with active exhalation, reduced lung volume, and breath holding with central apnea.[15]

$Paco_2$ and Pao_2 Orchestrate Ventilatory Responses

Maturation of central and peripheral arterial chemoreceptors will be briefly presented; please refer to article on the topic by Brown and Gauda[16] and narrative review by van der Heijden and Zoghbi[17] for a more comprehensive overview of central and peripheral mechanisms that control breathing during development.

Central chemoreceptors: CO_2/H^+, sensors: Breathing begins with rhythmogenesis, controlled by the pre-Bötzinger complex (preBötC) and the retrotrapezoid/parafacial nucleus (RTN/pF) in the brainstem. The preBötC produces respiratory rhythms, while the RTN, containing central chemoreceptors sensitive to CO_2/H^+, provides excitatory input to the preBötC. Their activity is closely linked and necessary to sustain ventilation after birth. Premature infants have a narrow CO_2 reserve, decreased Pco_2 chemosensitivity, and weak coupling between the preBotC and RTN, all contributing to unstable breathing.[18] Infants with congenital central hypoventilation syndrome have a genetic mutation in the Phox2B gene that compromises development of central chemoreceptors.[19] These infants often require ventilatory support or diaphragmatic pacing.[20]

Peripheral arterial chemoreceptors: O_2 sensors: The ventilatory response to oxygen is regulated by

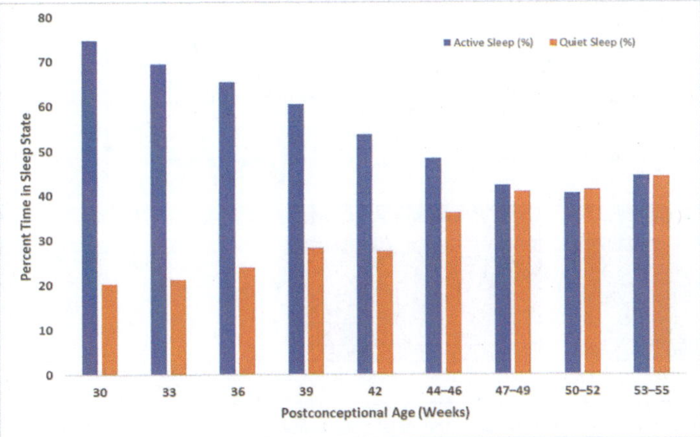

Fig. 1. Maturational trajectory of changes in active and quiet sleep in premature infants. (*Data from* Holditch-Davis D, Scher M, Schwartz T, et al. Sleeping and waking state development in preterm infants. Early Hum Dev. 2004.)

peripheral arterial chemoreceptors, which are highly sensitive and respond rapidly to changes in oxygen tension. After initial silencing at birth, chemoreceptor activity increases with maturation, causing periodic breathing. While the initial increase in ventilation in response to hypoxia is mediated by peripheral chemoreceptors, within seconds to minutes it is followed by respiratory depression that is secondary to central inhibition. The immature response to hypoxia is a greater reduction in ventilation often leading to apnea. This central[21] respiratory depression is from rapid metabolism of ATP to adenosine which inhibits ventilation by binding to adenosine receptors on respiratory related neurons.[21,22]

Conceptualizing Breathing Instability: Central Apnea and Periodic Breathing are the Expression of Loop Gain

As depicted in the schematic in **Fig. 2**, breathing stability is governed by loop gain, the propensity of the ventilatory control system to oscillate after a disturbance; a loop gain of greater than 1 breathing is unstable, characterized by apneas and periodic breathing, and loop gain less than 1 equates to breathing stability (see **Fig. 2**).[23,24] Several physiologic parameters determine loop gain, including the sensitivity of the central and peripheral chemoreceptors, lung capacity and compliance, and circulatory delay time (see **Fig. 2**). Loop gain is the product of controller gain and plant gain. Controller gain is the magnitude of the output from the central respiratory network in response to inputs from central and peripheral chemoreceptors—how much respiratory output from the brainstem increases ventilation for a given increase in $Paco_2$ or drop in Pao_2. Plant gain is determined by buffering capacity for CO_2 and O_2 in the lung (FRC) and the body (Hgb) and determines how much $Paco_2$ and Pao_2 change given a change in ventilation. Low levels of FRC will cause large swings in $Paco_2$ for a unit change in ventilation, destabilizing breathing. For example, low lung volumes trigger sighs (augmented breaths), that rapidly lowers $Paco_2$ and increase Pao_2, causing post-sigh apnea.[25] Reduced lung volumes and atelectasis promote CO_2 retention, triggering compensatory tachypnea that overshoots ventilation and further lowers $Paco_2$, perpetuating cycles of apnea and hyperpnea characteristic of periodic breathing in premature infants. Stressors such as sepsis can augment unstable breathing and can be an early marker of sepsis.[26] Please see Edwards and colleagues[23] for a more thorough discussion of loop-gain and breathing stability.

Treatment of Apnea of Prematurity: Targeting Loop Gain

Understanding the concept of loop gain and the physiologic components can guide therapy. As listed in **Table 1**, caffeine and continuous positive airway pressure (CPAP) lower loop gain are the most effective treatments for stabilizing breathing in premature infants. Caffeine increases central chemoreceptor sensitivity and blocks adenosine's inhibition of the respiratory network. CPAP raises FRC, which improves lung buffering capacity and reduces apnea, IH, and sighs. Supplemental oxygen also stabilizes breathing by reducing peripheral chemoreceptor activity and increasing oxygen reserves. Red blood cell transfusion transiently decreases apnea and IH events.[27,28]

Caffeine safety and efficacy: In premature infants $\leq$ 30 weeks of gestation at birth, caffeine reduces frequency of apnea and IH episodes, respiratory morbidities and improves short-term and long-term motor outcomes. Infants are given 10 to 20 mg/kg loading dose, then 5 to 10 mg/kg daily started within 3 days of birth and continued until 34 weeks PMA; this dosing regime was used

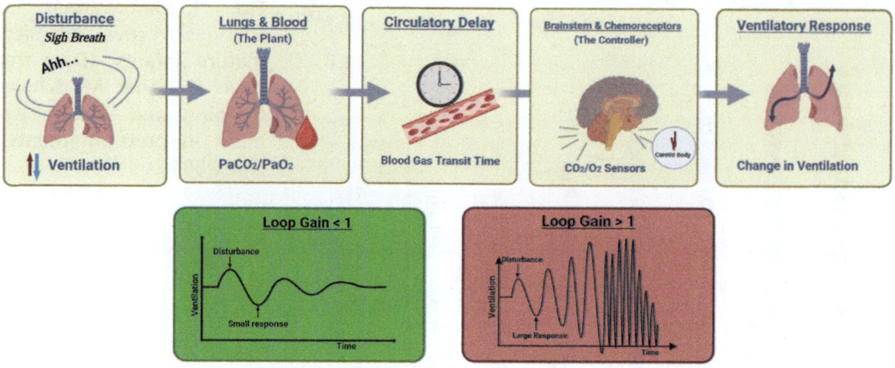

Loop gain is the ratio of the corrective response to the initial disturbance

Fig. 2. Schematic depicting the components of loop-gain: "plant (lung)" and controller (chemoreceptors) modulating breathing in premature infants. A disturbance (sigh breath) alters ventilation and blood gases, which are sensed after a circulatory delay by brainstem chemoreceptors to generate a corrective response. In premature infants, immature respiratory control, low lung volumes, and prolonged circulatory delay increase loop gain, predisposing to ventilatory instability, periodic breathing, and central apnea. (Created in BioRender. Antwi, J. (2026) https://BioRender.com/s6sdu2y.)

in the Caffeine for Apnea of Prematurity (CAP) trial RCT.[29] CPAP is commonly used in conjunction with caffeine. In most infants, caffeine can be safely discontinued at 33 weeks PMA after 7 days of being apneic free.[30,31] However, infants at increased risk of residual lung disease should be closely monitored for IH after stopping caffeine even at 34 weeks PMA,[32] and infants should be event free for 5 to 7 days prior to discharge. Of note, 10% to 30% of preterm infants have caffeine resistant apnea, and although higher doses of caffeine and different dosing strategies have been used and reported,[33] they are not recommended. Only the dosing strategy used in the CAP trial has been rigorously evaluated for short-term and long-term safety and efficacy.[34]

Doxapram enhancing hypoxic chemosensitivity: Doxapram is used for caffeine-refractory apnea to avoid intubation and is used more in Europe than in North America for this indication.[35] It increases carotid body hypoxic sensitivity and central respiratory drive without augmenting CO_2 chemosensitivity.[36] The ongoing DOXA trial (NCT004430790) a multicenter randomized trial is evaluating its safety and efficacy, with death or severe neurodevelopmental impairment at 18 to 24 months as the primary outcome.[37]

Table 1
Physiologic parameters that determine and therapies that modify loop gain in premature infants

Loop Gain Component	Physiologic Factors	Direction of Effect	Mechanism	Treatments	Effect on Loop Gain
Controller gain	Immature RTN/pFRG chemosensitivity	↓	Weak CO_2 response → apnea	Caffeine	↑ Controller gain
Controller gain	Hyper-reactive carotid bodies	↑	Overshoot ventilation	Supplemental O_2	↓ Peripheral gain
Plant gain	Low FRC	↑↑	Small gas reservoir → large ΔPCO_2	CPAP	↓ Plant gain
Plant gain	High metabolic rate	↑	Large CO_2 oscillations	Maturation	↓ Plant gain
Plant gain	Poor V/Q matching	↑	Gas-exchange instability	O_2, CPAP	↓ Plant gain
Feedback delay	Immature arousal mechanisms	↑	Delayed response to hypoventilation	Caffeine	↓ Effective delay

Consequences of Central Apnea and Intermittent Hypoxemia

Apnea and IH burden are greatest in the most immature premature infants and is associated with a higher risk of a range of morbidities including poor respiratory outcomes, neurodevelopmental impairment, and retinopathy of prematurity.[38–42] Recurrent IH increases oxidative stress that damages developing organs.[43] Although AoP typically resolves before hospital discharge, children born preterm remain at increased risk for disordered breathing in infancy and childhood.[44] This risk is primarily attributable to prematurity-related alterations in ventilatory control and airway development, rather than to the history of apnea. Former premature infants, regardless of apnea history, are more vulnerable to sleep-disordered breathing due to changes in the respiratory network and increased risk of sudden infant death syndrome and brief resolved unexplained events (BRUEs).[45] As reviewed in Gauda and colleagues, extrauterine environmental exposures during the last trimester of fetal development predisposes the infant to ineffective breathing responses to environmental stressors after birth.[46]

In summary, AoP occurs in almost all infants born $\leq$ 28 weeks of gestation and ~90% of the apnea that occur in premature infants have a central component. These infants have high loop gain due to immature lungs and respiratory control, increasing their risk of apnea, periodic breathing, and hypoxemia, which contributes to respiratory and neurologic comorbidities. Understanding the concept of loop gain and the physiologic components that control it can inform therapies to stabilize breathing. Caffeine continues to be the cornerstone of therapy, effectively targeting several components of loop gain to stabilize breathing. The efficacy of doxapram for caffeine failures is less well established. When pharmacotherapy fails, invasive ventilation may be necessary but is associated with worse outcomes. Additional research is needed to guide caffeine dosing in the smallest infants. Safe pharmacologic and nonpharmacological therapies that are efficacious are needed when caffeine fails.

CENTRAL APNEA IN INFANCY

Definition, Epidemiology

The AAP defines apnea of infancy as an unexplained episode of cessation of breathing lasting $\geq$20 seconds, or a shorter pause accompanied by bradycardia, cyanosis, pallor, and/or hypotonia, occurring in an infant beyond the neonatal period (generally >37 weeks postmenstrual age).[47,48] Polysomnography is used to accurately diagnosis apnea of infancy and according to the American Academy of Sleep Medicine (AASM) central apnea is scored when there is complete cessation of airflow with absent inspiratory effort lasting $\geq$20 seconds, or a shorter pause lasting at least 2 missed breaths when accompanied by an arousal, awakening, $\geq$3% oxygen desaturation, or bradycardia. A central apnea index (CAI) greater than 5 events/hour is commonly regarded as abnormal in term infants.[49]

Pathogenesis

Similar to AoP, delayed maturation of respiratory network and peripheral inputs that modify its activity is a common cause of central apnea of infancy. Although AoP usually resolves by 34 to 36 weeks post-menstrual age, apnea and bradycardia frequently persist beyond term in infants born at 24 to 28 weeks' gestation.[31,50] Former preterm infants continue to show delayed maturation of breathing regulation at term-equivalent age,[51] and very preterm infants evaluated at 12 to 15 months corrected age have attenuated ventilatory response to hypoxia.[52]

Primary central sleep apnea of infancy using American Academy of Paediatrics (AAP) criteria is defined as central apnea/desaturation, confirmed by polysomnography showing recurrent prolonged central apneas ($\geq$20 seconds) or periodic breathing $\geq$5% of sleep time in term or near-term infants with sleep-related central apneas and who otherwise have normal development. It is rare and a diagnosis of exclusion. It is benign and self-limited, with spontaneous resolution over the first year of life; management is largely supportive. Short-term caffeine therapy is reserved for infants with frequent or clinically significant events,[53] with a good therapeutic response reported for some infants.

Genetic Causes of Central Apnea of Infancy

Gene mutations, such as those in the PHOX2B gene, can disrupt respiratory network development and rhythmogenesis, leading to conditions like congenital central hypoventilation syndrome (CCHS). Infants with CCHS commonly experience recurrent apnea soon after birth due to reduced CO_2 chemoreceptor sensitivity and impaired autonomic functions. Disease severity varies based on mutation type and repeat number, with some infants needing nighttime-assisted ventilation and others requiring support during wakefulness.[19]

Infants with Trisomy 21 can have dysregulation of central respiratory control. They often have upper airway obstruction, but central apnea is also relatively common, particularly in younger children less than 2 years of age.[54] Central apnea may occur during sleep, after crying, or spontaneously, episodes may be brief and self-resolving while others may require stimulation or assisted ventilation. Chou and colleagues reported 27.5% apnea rate in Trisomy 21 infants $\leq$ 12 months.[55] Of note, central apnea improved after adenotonsillectomy in a cohort of infants with Trisomy 21.[56] Taira and colleagues reported that recurrent apnea was common in infants with Trisomy 18, likely due to immature brainstem circuits, upper-airway obstruction, or both. Disordered breathing in children with Trisomy 18 can mask co-existing seizures presenting as apnea that often respond to antiepileptic therapy.[57]

Prader–Willi syndrome results from loss of paternally expressed genes in the chromosome 15q11–q13 region, most commonly due to a paternal deletion, maternal uniparental disomy, or imprinting defect. These infants have central apnea and blunted ventilatory responses to hypoxia and hypercapnic ventilatory in addition to hypotonia, weak respiratory muscles, scoliosis, and obesity.[58] Rett syndrome is caused by an X-linked dominant mutation of the MECP2 gene and manifests with developmental, neurologic, and growth abnormalities emerging in the first year of life. Affected girls (boys rarely survive) have episodes of hyperventilation, breath-holding, and central apnea.[59]

Sepsis commonly suppresses respiratory drive in infants, with apnea as a frequent presenting sign.[60] Interleukin-1β (IL-1β) disrupts breathing by inducing prostaglandin E_2 (PGE_2), prolonging laryngeal apnea and impairing autoresuscitation in animal models, and higher IL-1β levels correlate with more severe central apnea in infants with respiratory syncytial viral (RSV) infection.[61,62] Mechanistically, IL-1β activates endothelial signaling at the blood–brain barrier, inducing COX-2 and mPGES-1 and increasing central PGE_2, which suppresses tidal volume and ventilatory responsiveness to CO_2.[63] Consistent with this pathway, neonates receiving exogenous PGE_2 to maintain ductal patency often develop respiratory depression; methylxanthines have been used to stimulate respiratory; aminophylline[64] may be more effective than caffeine.[65]

Bilirubin Encephalopathy: Respiratory instability, including apnea and periodic breathing, can be among the early neurologic signs in infants who develop bilirubin encephalopathy, particularly in preterm or critically ill neonates.[66] Unconjugated bilirubin crosses the immature blood–brain barrier and deposits in regions of high metabolic activity, including respiratory-related brainstem nuclei controlling respiration.[67]

Seizure presenting as apnea: Ictal apnea is a seizure-related cessation of breathing resulting from transient suppression of central respiratory control and may be the sole clinical manifestation of seizures in infants.[68] In this age group, episodes typically present as sudden central apnea with oxygen desaturation and bradycardia, often without overt motor activity, and are recurrent and stereotyped. Diagnosis requires simultaneous video-EEG with cardiorespiratory monitoring demonstrating electrographic seizure activity temporally linked to apnea. Ictal apnea must be distinguished from BRUE and apnea of infancy as management requires prompt identification and treatment of the underlying seizure disorder. BRUE and apnea of infancy would not have corresponding EEG changes with cessation of breathing.

Exogenous Respiratory Depressants

Maternal drug exposure can suppress fetal and neonatal respiration. Opioids, used by 1 in 20 pregnant women, may decrease neonatal respiratory drive and increase the need for support after birth.[69] Prenatal opioid exposure disrupts brainstem respiratory networks, reducing rhythm stability and heightening postnatal opioid-related respiratory depression.[70] Late pregnancy benzodiazepine exposure leads to neonatal hypotonia and respiratory depression.[71] Serotonin uptake inhibitors are increasingly used during pregnancy; while apnea and respiratory depression are uncommon, it has been reported in one infant exposed to high-dose sertraline throughout pregnancy.[72] Thorough review of maternal medications, peripartum analgesics, and neonatal drug exposures is crucial when assessing central apnea in healthy term infants at birth.

Brainstem Compression from Structural Defects

Mechanical narrowing or distortion at the craniocervical junction can compromise brainstem respiratory pathways, resulting in central apnea.[73] In infants with achondroplasia, foramen stenosis and Chiari-like malformations may cause both central and obstructive apneas, though symptoms do not always correlate with foramen magnum size, indicating possible central dysfunction without severe narrowing.[74] Both types of apnea often improve after foramen magnum decompression.[75] Based on an international consensus statement,[76] routine screening for sleep-disordered breathing with polysomnography should be done for all infants with achondroplasia, and expert opinion suggests similar monitoring for those with Chiari malformation because of the risk for brainstem compression.

Laryngeal Chemoreflex-Induced Apnea

Laryngeal stimulation in infants triggers central apnea, and the magnitude of response is substantially more pronounced during mild hypoxia,[77] and in premature infants.[78] Refluxate from the stomach reaching the larynx can stimulate the laryngeal chemoreflex, triggering apnea, laryngeal closure, or bradycardia.[79] Some have suggested reflux could contribute to severe apnea or even sudden infant death syndrome in term infants.[80] However, gastroesophageal reflux (GER) and apnea are common in premature infants, but GER does not cause apnea in premature infants.[81]

Consequences of Severe Apnea: Sudden Infant Death Syndrome

The ultimate apnea is the one from which the infant does not recover, leading to death. Sudden infant death syndrome (SIDS) refers to the unexplained death of an infant under 12 months that remains unresolved after thorough investigation.[82] The triple-risk model suggests SIDS occurs when a vulnerable infant faces an external stressor during a critical period.[83] Impaired arousal and brainstem respiratory regulation, observed in infants with central apnea, are observed in infants who later died of SIDS (Kato I and Franco P, 2003). Prone sleeping reduces arousal response to obstructive apneas, possibly prolonging central apneas. Abnormalities in medullary serotonin pathways affect ventilatory drive and arousal in infants who died from SIDS.[84] While central apnea has intrinsic causes, factors like sleep environment and exposure to smoke or alcohol can raise vulnerability.[85] Promoting supine sleeping through the Back to Sleep campaign has significantly reduced SIDS rates.[86]

Evaluation and Management of Central Apnea in Infancy

Many infants and children with central apnea may be asymptomatic, underscoring the importance of targeted polysomnography screening in high-risk groups.[87] Polysomnography remains the gold standard for diagnosing central and obstructive apnea and nocturnal hypoventilation in children and must be interpreted using age-specific norms.[88]

When central sleep apnea is identified in an otherwise healthy infant, neuroimaging is recommended, with additional testing guided by clinical context. Management depends on the underlying condition and symptom burden; medically complex children—including those with Down syndrome, Prader–Willi syndrome, neuromuscular disorders, congenital heart disease, achondroplasia, or Arnold–Chiari malformation—often require multidisciplinary care.[87]

Treatment varies by pathophysiology. Self-limited immaturity of respiratory control is typically managed with observation, while low-flow oxygen may benefit select infants.[53] Identifiable neurologic, metabolic, or structural disorders require targeted therapy, and pharmacologic agents may be considered in select cases.

In summary, central apnea of infancy occurs 1 per 1000 infants born at term which should be diagnosed with polysomnography, using objective criteria. The pathogenesis often involves delayed maturation of respiratory control, especially in former preterm infants, though it can also be due to rare, self-limited primary central sleep apnea, genetic conditions (such as PHOX2B mutations, Trisomy 21 or 18, Prader–Willi, and Rett syndromes), infections like sepsis, bilirubin encephalopathy, seizures, exposure to respiratory depressants, or brainstem compression from anatomic abnormalities. Evaluation should include polysomnography and, in some cases, neuroimaging and a multidisciplinary approach. Management depends on the underlying cause, with many cases resolving spontaneously, while others require targeted therapies or supportive interventions based on specific diagnoses.

DETECTING CENTRAL APNEA

The National Institutes of Health (NIH) and AAP guidelines define apnea as a cessation of flow for $\geq$ 20 seconds or a shorter respiratory pause associated with bradycardia, cyanosis, pallor, or marked hypotonia.[2,89] Events are categorized as central (no flow and lack of respiratory efforts), obstructive (respiratory efforts with no flow), and mixed (events that contain both central and obstructive components). Central AoP is common in extremely preterm infants, increasing in frequency during the first month of life with the number of events decreasing with increasing gestational age at birth.[1] Apnea of infancy occurs in infants $\geq$ 37 weeks of gestation through the first year of life. It is diagnosed using polysomnography; central apnea is scored when there is complete cessation of airflow with absent inspiratory effort lasting $\geq$20 seconds, or a shorter pause lasting at least 2 missed breaths when accompanied by an arousal, awakening, $\geq$3% oxygen desaturation, or bradycardia. A CAI greater than 5 events/hour is abnormal in term infants.[49] Accurate detection of apnea continues to be a challenge in the clinical environment, relying on both quantitative and qualitative measures of flow or volume.

Pneumotachometer the gold standard: The pneumotachometer is the gold standard for measuring flow and volume but must be incorporated into a sealed nasal/oral mask or attached to an endotracheal tube. It also may add a significant resistive load, especially in severely ill patients. As a result, many companies have pivoted to a hot-wire anemometer for volume measures during mechanical ventilation due to its high-frequency response, lower resistive load, and proven accuracy.

Detecting Apnea in Premature Infants in the Neonatal Intensive Care Unit

Impedance monitoring remains the primary technology for measuring respiration in the neonatal intensive care unit. Transthoracic impedance monitoring employs a small electrical current between 2 chest electrodes. As the infant chest wall expands and contracts with each breath, the distance between the electrodes changes with corresponding alterations in the body's electrical impedance. Measures of impedance are then converted to a respiratory rate using proprietary waveform algorithms. Ideally, these algorithms should be capable of identifying central respiratory pauses, even when masked by motion artifact or occurring alongside obstructed efforts. This is particularly challenging during obstructed breaths, as air moves from one lung compartment to another, causing these respiratory efforts to be mistaken for normal respiration. Transthoracic impedance also tends to miss breaths during motion or following large sighs with overall poor sensitivity in identifying central apnea.[90,91]

Respiratory inductance plethysmography: Pneumograms and polysomnograms used for diagnosis and thus require more accurate detection of respiration and the ability to detect both central and obstructive apnea. Respiratory inductance plethysmography uses 2 bands around the chest and abdomen. As the chest wall expands, the coils in the bands elongate altering the magnetic properties, or inductance, of each band. These alterations provide a 2-dimensional representation of volume in the abdominal and chest wall compartments allowing for identification of central apnea and distinction of synchronous from asynchronous breathing. The integration of software providing a semiquantitative “sum” or nasal/oral flow sensors (eg, thermistor, end tidal CO_2) facilitates the detection of obstructive apnea during periods of asynchronous respiratory efforts.

Neurally adjusted ventilatory assist: Other technologies include neurally adjusted ventilatory assist that provides neural measures of electrical diaphragmatic activity to identify apnea and provide synchronized support during mechanical ventilation.[92] In crossover trials, neurally adjusted ventilatory assist improved oxygenation and reduced work of breathing.[93] Similar support can be performed during noninvasive ventilation via changes in pneumatic pressure from a capsule placed on the abdomen. Recent data in a small cohort of extremely preterm infants showed significant improvement in apnea detection when compared to conventional impedance monitoring.[90]

Artificial intelligence with the inevitable application of artificial intelligence in neonatal care, there has been increased interest in development of new data analytics to improve apnea identification. In the research setting, employment of cardiac filtering has been shown to reduce the chance of heart beats being mistaken for respiration,[94] especially during periods of bradycardia.[95] Stochastic models have analyzed the distribution of duration and time between apnea to predict the frequency of prolonged events during the first year of life,[96] and machine learning techniques have improved automated central detection,[97] with a reduction in false alarm events.[98] Application of wavelet transform methods has allowed quantification of periodic breathing, a cyclical pattern of short apneic pauses and breaths that are often accompanied by desaturation.[99]

Pulse Oximetry: Due to the limited performance of thoracic impedance monitoring in identifying apnea, infant monitoring commonly includes pulse oximetry and electrocardiography. Pulse oximetry has become a major contributor in identifying infants with oxygenation instability that can accompany respiratory pauses with studies consistently showing a relationship between intermittent hypoxic events and a range of sequelae including retinopathy of prematurity,[38,100] neurodevelopmental impairment,[100,101] and bronchopulmonary dysplasia.[39,102]

Machine Learning and Predictive Analytics: Models such as Shannon entropy and Kalman filter applications, among others, have leveraged the addition of heart rate or oxygen saturation time series, employing correlations with heart rate, respiratory rate, and SpO_2, enhancing automated detection of apnea.[103–105] Machine learning applications have also yielded tools for disease prediction in preterm infants. For example, a significantly higher number of central apnea was noted in the 6-hour window prior to sepsis onset.[106] Recent large trials including apnea, hypoxemia, and bradycardia have found a significant increase in relative risk of late onset sepsis with overall prolonged periods of IH and dynamic increases in apnea, periodic breathing, and bradycardia in the day preceding sepsis diagnosis.[26] Even cardiorespiratory events with mild decreases in SpO_2 are associated with increased risk of bronchopulmonary dysplasia and prolonged need for respiratory support.[40,107] Many of these machine learning approaches have potential for identifying apnea at the bedside and infants at risk for both short-term and long-term morbidity. However, larger cohort studies with external validation are needed to assess generalizability, including effects of maturation and illness severity. Lastly, ethical concerns—such as accountability for misdiagnosis or event detection, along with cost analyses—must be addressed before integrating AI models into clinical practice.

CLINICS CARE POINTS

- Polysomnography is the gold standard for assessing and characterizing central apnea in term infants.
- Gastroesophageal reflux is an uncommon cause of recurrent central apneas in premature infants, and routine anti-reflux therapy should not be used.
- Caffeine is the first-line therapy for apnea of prematurity. It reduces signficant apnea, facilitates extubation, decreases bronchopulmonary dysplasia and is associated with improved neurodevelopment outcomes.
- Stopping caffeine should be individualized and guided by postmenstrual age, event-free interval, respiratory support, gestational age at birth and risk for persistent intermittent hypoxic events.

ACKNOWLEDGMENTS

The authors would like to thank Douglas Watson, MD, for copy editing the manuscript and his helpful suggestions, Ms Sonia dos Santos for her exceptional administrative assistance, and Mr Jeffry Antwi for creating the figures.

DISCLOSURE

The authors have nothing to disclose.

FUNDING

The work was fundedby the Women's Auxiliary Chair in Neonatology, The Hospital for Sick Children, The SickKids Foundation.

REFERENCES

1. Weese-Mayer DE, Di Fiore JM, Lake DE, et al. Maturation of cardioventilatory physiological trajectories in extremely preterm infants. Pediatr Res 2024;95(4):1060–9.
2. Eichenwald EC, Watterberg KL, Aucott S, et al. Apnea of prematurity. Pediatrics 2016;137(1).
3. Patel M, Mohr M, Lake D, et al. Clinical associations with immature breathing in preterm infants: part 2—periodic breathing. Pediatr Res 2016; 80(1):28–34.
4. Glotzbach SF, Baldwin RB, Lederer NE, et al. Periodic breathing in preterm infants: incidence and characteristics. Pediatrics 1989;84(5):785–92.
5. Mathew OP, Roberts JL, Thach BT. Pharyngeal airway obstruction in preterm infants during mixed and obstructive apnea. J Pediatr 1982;100(6):964–8.
6. Strohl KP, Hensley MJ, Hallett M, et al. Activation of upper airway muscles before onset of inspiration in normal humans. J Appl Physiol 1980;49(4):638–42.
7. Carlo WA, Martin RJ, Abboud EF, et al. Effect of sleep state and hypercapnia on alae nasi and diaphragm EMGs in preterm infants. J Appl Physiol 1983;54(6):1590–6.
8. Gauda EB, Miller MJ, Carlo WA, et al. Genioglossus and diaphragm activity during obstructive apnea and airway occlusion in infants. Pediatr Res 1989;26(6):583–4.
9. Di Fiore JM, Martin RJ, Gauda EB. Apnea of prematurity – perfect storm. Respir Physiol Neurobiol 2013;189(2):213–22.
10. Holditch-Davis D, Scher M, Schwartz T, et al. Sleeping and waking state development in preterm infants. Early Hum Dev 2004;80(1):43–64.
11. Holditch-Davis D, Scher M, Schwartz T. Respiratory development in preterm infants. J Perinatol 2004; 24(10):631–9.
12. Plunkett G, Yiallourou S, Voigt A, et al. Short apneas and periodic breathing in preterm infants in the neonatal intensive care unit—Effects of sleep position, sleep state, and age. J Sleep Res 2025; 34(1):e14253.
13. Schulte FJ, Busse C, Eichhorn W. Rapid eye movement sleep, motoneurone inhibition, and apneic spells in preterm infants. Pediatr Res 1977;11(6):709–13.
14. Hardman JG, Wills JS, Aitkenhead AR. Factors determining the onset and course of hypoxemia during apnea: an investigation using physiological modelling. Anesth Analg 2000;90(3):619–24.
15. Dormishian A, Schott A, Aguilar AC, et al. Etiology and mechanism of intermittent hypoxemia episodes in spontaneously breathing extremely premature infants. J Pediatr 2023;262:113623.
16. Brown A, Tamir Hostovsky L, Gauda EB. Developmental changes in the respiratory system of the neonate-child. In: Chowdhuri SM, Badr S, Rowley JA,

editors. Control of breathing during sleep. 1st edition. Boca Raton (FL): CRC Press; 2022.
17. van der Heijden ME, Zoghbi HY. Development of the brainstem respiratory circuit. WIREs Dev Biol 2020;9(3):e366.
18. Moriette G, Van Reempts P, Moore M, et al. The effect of rebreathing CO2 on ventilation and diaphragmatic electromyography in newborn infants. Respir Physiol 1985;62(3):387–97.
19. Kasi AS, Perez IA. Congenital central hypoventilation syndrome and disorders of control of ventilation. Clin Chest Med 2024;45(3):663–73.
20. Marion TL, Bradshaw WT. Congenital central hypoventilation syndrome and the *PHOX2B* gene mutation. Neonatal Network 2011;30(6):397–401.
21. Yan S, Laferriere A, Zhang C, et al. Microdialyzed adenosine in nucleus tractus solitarii and ventilatory response to hypoxia in piglets. J Appl Physiol 1995;79(2):405–10.
22. Koos BJ. Adenosine A 2a receptors and O 2 sensing in development. Am J Physiol Regul Integr Comp Physiol 2011;301(3):R601–22.
23. Edwards BA, Sands SA, Berger PJ. Postnatal maturation of breathing stability and loop gain: the role of carotid chemoreceptor development. Respir Physiol Neurobiol 2013;185(1):144–55.
24. Javaheri S, Badr MS. Central sleep apnea: pathophysiologic classification. Sleep 2023;46(3):zsac113.
25. Severs LJ, Vlemincx E, Ramirez JM. The psychophysiology of the sigh: I: the sigh from the physiological perspective. Biol Psychol 2022;170:108313.
26. Kausch SL, Lake DE, Di Fiore JM, et al. Apnea, intermittent hypoxemia, and bradycardia events predict late-onset sepsis in infants born extremely preterm. J Pediatr 2024;271:114042.
27. Joshi A, Gerhardt T, Shandloff P, et al. Blood transfusion effect on the respiratory pattern of preterm infants. Pediatrics 1987;80(1):79–84.
28. Abu Jawdeh EG, Martin RJ, Dick TE, et al. The effect of red blood cell transfusion on intermittent hypoxemia in ELBW infants. J Perinatol 2014;34(12):921–5.
29. Schmidt B, Roberts RS, Davis P, et al. Caffeine therapy for apnea of prematurity. N Engl J Med 2006;354(20):2112–21.
30. Prakash R, Pournami F, Prabhakar J, et al. Duration of caffeine for apnea of prematurity - a randomized controlled trial. Indian J Pediatr 2021;88(12):1174–9.
31. Lorch SA, Srinivasan L, Escobar GJ. Epidemiology of apnea and bradycardia resolution in premature infants. Pediatrics 2011;128(2):e366–73.
32. Mashep PK, Ochieng R, Coleman J, et al. Impact of cessation of caffeine citrate therapy on intermittent hypoxemia patterns among preterm infants born before 34 weeks. Front Pediatr 2025;13:1463484.
33. Saroha V, Patel RM. Caffeine for preterm infants: fixed standard dose, adjustments for age or high dose? Semin Fetal Neonatal Med 2020;25(6):101178.
34. Schmidt B. Caffeine for apnea of prematurity: too much or too little of a good thing. J Pediatr 2023;259:113488.
35. Lavizzari A, Hutten GJ, Heiring C, et al. Management of apnoea in extremely preterm infants: a European Survey. Neonatology 2025;122(6):677–84.
36. Yost CS. A new look at the respiratory stimulant doxapram. CNS Drug Rev 2006;12(3–4):236–49.
37. Poppe JA, Flint RB, Smits A, et al. Doxapram versus placebo in preterm newborns: a study protocol for an international double blinded multicentre randomized controlled trial (DOXA-trial). Trials 2023;24(1):656.
38. Di Fiore JM, Kaffashi F, Loparo K, et al. The relationship between patterns of intermittent hypoxia and retinopathy of prematurity in preterm infants. Pediatr Res 2012;72(6):606–12.
39. Jensen EA, Whyte RK, Schmidt B, et al. Association between intermittent hypoxemia and severe bronchopulmonary dysplasia in preterm infants. Am J Respir Crit Care Med 2021;204(10):1192–9.
40. Ambalavanan N, Weese-Mayer DE, Hibbs AM, et al. Cardiorespiratory monitoring data to predict respiratory outcomes in extremely preterm infants. Am J Respir Crit Care Med 2023;208(1):79–97.
41. Poets CF. Intermittent hypoxia and long-term neurological outcome: how are they related? Semin Fetal Neonatal Med 2020;25(2):101072.
42. Kim F, Bateman DA, Garey D, et al. Association between intermittent hypoxemia and neurodevelopmental outcomes in extremely premature infants: a single-center experience. Early Hum Dev 2024;188:105919.
43. Thompson L, Werthammer JW, Gozal D. Apnea of prematurity and oxidative stress: potential implications. Antioxidants 2024;13(11):1304.
44. Crump C, Friberg D, Li X, et al. Preterm birth and risk of sleep-disordered breathing from childhood into mid-adulthood. Int J Epidemiol 2019;48(6):2039–49.
45. Horne RSC, Harrewijn I, Hunt CE. Physiology during sleep in preterm infants: implications for increased risk for the sudden infant death syndrome. Sleep Med Rev 2024;78:101990.
46. Gauda EB, McLemore GL. Premature birth, homeostatic plasticity and respiratory consequences of inflammation. Respir Physiol Neurobiol 2020;274:103337.
47. Committee on Fetus and Newborn. American Academy of Pediatrics. Apnea, sudden infant death syndrome, and home monitoring. Pediatrics 2003;111(4 Pt 1):914–7.

48. Engle W, American Academy of Pediatrics Committee on Fetus and Newborn. Age terminology during the perinatal period. Pediatrics 2004;114(5):1362–4.
49. Berry R, Quan S, Abreu A. The AASM manual for the scoring of sleep and associated events: rules, terminology and technical specifications, version 2.6. Darien: American Academy of Sleep Medicine; 2020.
50. Eichenwald EC, Aina A, Stark AR. Apnea frequently persists beyond term gestation in infants delivered at 24 to 28 weeks. Pediatrics 1997;100(3):354–9.
51. Erickson G, Dobson NR, Hunt CE. Immature control of breathing and apnea of prematurity: the known and unknown. J Perinatol 2021;41(9):2111–23.
52. Freislich Z, Stoecklin B, Hemy N, et al. The ventilatory response to hypoxia is blunted in some preterm infants during the second year of life. Front Pediatr 2022;10:974643.
53. Hayashi A, Suresh S, Kevat A, et al. Central sleep apnea in otherwise healthy term infants. J Clin Sleep Med 2022;18(12):2813–7.
54. Naime S, Weiss M, Lew J, et al. Central breathing abnormalities in children with trisomy 21: effect of age, sex, and concomitant OSA. Pediatr Pulmonol 2021;56(2):472–8.
55. Cho Y, Kwon Y, Ruth C, et al. The burden of sleep disordered breathing in infants with Down syndrome referred to tertiary sleep center. Pediatr Pulmonol 2023;58(4):1122–6.
56. Thottam PJ, Choi S, Simons JP, et al. Effect of adenotonsillectomy on central and obstructive sleep apnea in children with Down Syndrome. Otolaryngol Head Neck Surg 2015;153(4):644–8.
57. Taira R, Inoue H, Sawano T, et al. Management of apnea in infants with trisomy 18. Dev Med Child Neurol 2020;62(7):874–8.
58. Gillett E, Perez I. Disorders of sleep and ventilatory control in Prader-Willi Syndrome. Diseases 2016; 4(3):23.
59. Ramirez JM, Karlen-Amarante M, Wang JDJ, et al. Breathing disturbances in Rett syndrome. Handb Clin Neurol 2022;189:139–51.
60. Sangsari R, Saeedi M, Mirnia K, et al. A comparison of clinical and laboratory features in neonatal proven sepsis and COVID-19. Pediatr Infect Dis J 2025;44(4):351–6.
61. Lindgren C, Grögaard J. Reflex apnoea response and inflammatory mediators in infants with respiratory tract infection. Acta Paediatr 1996;85(7): 798–803.
62. Stoltenberg L, Sundar T, Almaas R, et al. Changes in apnea and autoresuscitation in piglets after intravenous and intrathecal interleukin-1β injection. jpme 1994;22(5):421–32.
63. Engblom D, Ek M, Saha S, et al. Prostaglandins as inflammatory messengers across the blood-brain barrier. J Mol Med 2002;80(1):5–15.
64. Lim DS, Kulik TJ, Kim DW, et al. Aminophylline for the prevention of apnea during prostaglandin E1 infusion. Pediatrics 2003;112(1):e27–9.
65. Salamati L, Dehghan B, Sabri MR, et al. Caffeine treatment for prostaglandin E1–Induced apnea prevention in congenital heart disease neonates: a randomized clinical trial. Crit Care Res Pract 2025;2025(1):4923280.
66. Watchko JF. Bilirubin-induced neurotoxicity in the preterm neonate. Clin Perinatol 2016;43(2): 297–311.
67. Amin SB, Bhutani VK, Watchko JF. Apnea in acute bilirubin encephalopathy. Semin Perinatol 2014; 38(7):407–11.
68. Falsaperla R, Consentino MC, Vitaliti G, et al. Isolated ictal apnea in neonatal age: clinical features and treatment options. A systematic review. Auton Neurosci 2022;243:103034.
69. Fältmarch S, Perttilä I, Tuomi U, et al. Use of opioids during pregnancy and effects of pregnancy outcomes. Pharmacoepidemiol Drug Saf 2019; 28(9):1239–45.
70. Beyeler SA, Naidoo R, Morrison NR, et al. Maternal opioids age-dependently impair neonatal respiratory control networks. Front Physiol 2023;14: 1109754.
71. Swortfiguer D, Cissoko H, Giraudeau B, et al. Retentissement néonatal de l'exposition aux benzodiazépines en fin de grossesse. Arch Pediatr 2005; 12(9):1327–31.
72. Marchand GJ, Meassick K, Wolf H, et al. Respiratory depression in a neonate born to mother on maximum dose sertraline: a case report. J Med Case Rep 2021;15(1):88.
73. Pauli RM, Horton VK, Glinski LP, et al. Prospective assessment of risks for cervicomedullary-junction compression in infants with achondroplasia. Am J Hum Genet 1995;56(3):732–44.
74. Ednick M, Tinkle BT, Phromchairak J, et al. Sleep-related respiratory abnormalities and arousal pattern in achondroplasia during early infancy. J Pediatr 2009;155(4):510–5.e1.
75. Kumagai N, Ogiwara H, Iwama T, et al. Sleep apnea in patients with achondroplasia associated with foramen magnum stenosis. J Neurosurg Pediatr 2025;36(3):353–9.
76. Savarirayan R, Ireland P, Irving M, et al. International consensus statement on the diagnosis, multidisciplinary management and lifelong care of individuals with achondroplasia. Nat Rev Endocrinol 2022;18(3):173–89.
77. Wennergren G, Hertzberg T, Milerad J, et al. Hypoxia reinforces laryngeal reflex bradycardia in infants. Acta Paediatr 1989;78(1):11–7.
78. Davies AM, Koenig JS, Thach BT. Upper airway chemoreflex responses to saline and water in preterm infants. J Appl Physiol 1988;64(4):1412–20.

79. Thach BT. Reflux associated apnea in infants. Am J Med 1997;103(5):120S–4S.
80. Thach BT. Sudden infant death syndrome: can gastroesophageal reflux cause sudden infant death? Am J Med 2000;108(4):144–8.
81. Di Fiore JM, Arko M, Whitehouse M, et al. Apnea is not prolonged by acid gastroesophageal reflux in preterm infants. Pediatrics 2005;116(5):1059–63.
82. Ramirez JM, Ramirez S, Anderson TM. Sudden infant death syndrome, sleep, and the physiology and pathophysiology of the respiratory network. In: Byard RW, Duncan JR, editors. SIDS sudden infant and early childhood death: the past, the present and the future. Adelaide, South Australia, Australia: University of Adelaide Press; 2018. p. 615–40.
83. Filiano JJ, Kinney HC. A perspective on neuropathologic findings in victims of the sudden infant death syndrome: the triple-risk model. Neonatology 1994; 65(3–4):194–7.
84. Kinney HC, Richerson GB, Dymecki SM, et al. The brainstem and serotonin in the sudden infant death syndrome. Annu Rev Pathol 2009;4(1):517–50.
85. Moon RY, Darnall RA, Feldman-Winter L, et al. SIDS and other sleep-related infant deaths: updated 2016 recommendations for a safe infant sleeping environment. Pediatrics 2016;138(5):e20162938.
86. Vennemann M, Fischer D, Jorch G, et al. Prevention of sudden infant death syndrome (SIDS) due to an active health monitoring system 20 years prior to the public "Back to Sleep" campaigns. Arch Dis Child 2006;91(4):324–6.
87. McLaren AT, Bin-Hasan S, Narang I. Diagnosis, management and pathophysiology of central sleep apnea in children. Paediatr Respir Rev 2019;30: 49–57.
88. Daftary AS, Jalou HE, Shively L, et al. Polysomnography reference values in healthy newborns. J Clin Sleep Med 2019;15(03):437–43.
89. National Institutes of Health Consensus Development. Conference on infantile apnea and home monitoring, Sept 29 to Oct 1, 1986. Pediatrics 1987;79(2):292–9.
90. Lim K, Eastwood-Sutherland C, Marshall AP, et al. Limitations of thoracic impedance monitoring for central apnoea detection in preterm infants. Acta Paediatr 2021;110(9):2550–2.
91. Brouillette RT, Morrow AS, Weese-Mayer DE, et al. Comparison of respiratory inductive plethysmography and thoracic impedance for apnea monitoring. J Pediatr 1987;111(3):377–83.
92. García-Muñoz Rodrigo F, Urquía Martí L, Galán Henríquez G, et al. Neural breathing patterns in preterm newborns supported with non-invasive neurally adjusted ventilatory assist. J Perinatol 2018;38(9):1235–41.
93. Kuitunen I, Rannankari M, Räsänen K. Neurally adjusted ventilatory assist (NAVA) in neonatal and pediatric critical care—A scoping review of randomized controlled trials. Pediatr Pulmonol 2025; 60(1):e21525.
94. Lee H, Rusin CG, Lake DE, et al. A new algorithm for detecting central apnea in neonates. Physiol Meas 2012;33(1):1–17.
95. Southall DP, Richards JM, Lau KC, et al. An explanation for failure of impedance apnoea alarm systems. Arch Dis Child 1980;55(1):63–5.
96. Clark MT, Delos JB, Lake DE, et al. Stochastic modeling of central apnea events in preterm infants. Physiol Meas 2016;37(4):463–84.
97. Shirwaikar RD, Acharya UD, Makkithaya K, et al. Optimizing neural networks for medical data sets: a case study on neonatal apnea prediction. Artif Intell Med 2019;98:59–76.
98. Varisco G, Peng Z, Kommers D, et al. Central apnea detection in premature infants using machine learning. Comput Methods Programs Biomed 2022;226:107155.
99. Mohr MA, Fairchild KD, Patel M, et al. Quantification of periodic breathing in premature infants. Physiol Meas 2015;36(7):1415–27.
100. Poets CF, Roberts RS, Schmidt B, et al. Association between intermittent hypoxemia or bradycardia and late death or disability in extremely preterm infants. JAMA 2015;314(6):595.
101. Di Fiore JM, Wilson-Costello D, Chen Z, et al. Intermittent hypoxemia and neurodevelopmental impairment at 12 and 24 months in preterm infants. Neonatology 2025;122(4):388–97.
102. Raffay TM, Dylag AM, Sattar A, et al. Neonatal intermittent hypoxemia events are associated with diagnosis of bronchopulmonary dysplasia at 36 weeks postmenstrual age. Pediatr Res 2019;85(3): 318–23.
103. Belal SY, Emmerson AJ, Beatty PCW. Automatic detection of apnoea of prematurity. Physiol Meas 2011;32(5):523–42.
104. Vergales B, Paget-Brown A, Lee H, et al. Accurate automated apnea analysis in preterm infants. Am J Perinatol 2013;31(02):157–62.
105. Montazeri GN, Shamsollahi MB, Ge D, et al. Apnea bradycardia detection based on new coupled hidden semi Markov model. Med Biol Eng Comput 2021;59(1):1–11.
106. Varisco G, Kommers D, Long X, et al. Optimized detection of central apneas preceding late-onset sepsis in premature infants. In: Guiraud D, Tong S, Bonato P, Lee SI, editors. 2021 43rd annual international conference of the IEEE engineering in medicine & biology society (EMBC). Mexico: IEEE; 2021. p. 5463–8.
107. Poets CF, Nelin L. Predicting pulmonary outcomes in extremely preterm infants from recordings of cardiorespiratory data: a question of chicken and egg. Am J Respir Crit Care Med 2023;208(1):11–2.

Central Sleep Apnea and Hypoventilation Disorders in Children

Indra Narang, BMedSci, MBBCH, MD[a,*], Chun Ting Au, RPSGT, PhD[b], Maida Lynn Chen, MD[c]

KEYWORDS

• Central hypoventilation • Sleep-disordered breathing • ROHHAD syndrome • Central sleep apnea • Ventilation • Diaphragm pacing • Pediatric

KEY POINTS

- Central sleep apnea and hypoventilation in children stem from disorders affecting brainstem or ventilatory control, requiring polysomnogram diagnosis, targeted interventions, and ongoing follow-up to manage.
- Central sleep apnea in children is frequently underdiagnosed due to nonspecific symptoms. Careful monitoring is needed to understand its long-term course and outcomes.
- Congenital Central Hypoventilation Syndrome is a rare *PHOX2b*-related disorder causing lifelong ventilatory dependence and multisystem dysautonomias, with severity linked to genotype and requiring multidisciplinary care.
- In ROHHAD syndrome, central sleep apnea and hypoventilation often develop progressively after rapid-onset obesity and hypothalamic dysfunction, often leading to severe respiratory instability.
- In Prader-Willi Syndrome, central sleep apnea and hypoventilation are common in infancy due to hypotonia, brainstem immaturity, and hypothalamic dysfunction, requiring early recognition and management.

CENTRAL SLEEP APNEA

Background

Central sleep apnea (CSA) is a sleep-related breathing disorder which occurs when there is diminished or absent respiratory effort. CSA is often associated with arterial oxygen desaturation, arousals, frequent nocturnal awakenings, and sleep fragmentation.[1] CSA may be a distinct phenomenon or co-exist with hypoventilation syndromes. CSA, as discussed here, is distinguished from apnea of prematurity (AOP), which is a clinical diagnosis of central apneas that last for 20 seconds and are accompanied by bradycardia and/or oxygen desaturations in infants born less than 37 weeks.[2] Virtually all infants less than 28 weeks have AOP, but this decreases to less than 20% at 34 weeks and less than 10% beyond 34 weeks.[2] Henceforth, CSA disorders beyond prematurity will be the focus of discussion.

In the pediatric population, the American Academy of Sleep Medicine (AASM) defines a central apnea as the absence of chest and/or abdominal movement associated with a cessation of airflow for more than 20 seconds or lasting more than 2 baseline respiratory cycles if it is associated with an arousal, an awakening, or an oxygen desaturation of at least 3%.[3] Alternative criteria in infants

[a] Department of Pediatrics, The Hospital for Sick Children, 175 Elizabeth Street, Toronto, Ontario, M5G 2G3, Canada; [b] Translational Medicine, Research Institute, The Hospital for Sick Children, 686 Bay Street, Toronto, Ontario, M5G 0A4, Canada; [c] Pulmonary and Sleep Division, Seattle Children's Hospital, University of Washington School of Medicine, 4800 Sand Point Way NE, Seattle, WA 98105, USA
* Corresponding author.
E-mail address: indra.narang@sickkids.ca

Sleep Med Clin 21 (2026) 377–396
https://doi.org/10.1016/j.jsmc.2026.05.004
1556-407X/26/

Abbreviations	
AASM	American Academy of Sleep Medicine
ANS	autonomic nervous system
AOP	apnea of prematurity
CA	central apnea
CCHS	congenital central hypoventilation syndrome
CH	central hypoventilation
CM	Chiari malformation
CPAP	continuous positive airway pressure
CSA	central sleep apnea
DP	diaphragm pacing
ICSD	International Classification of Sleep Disorder
LS	Leigh syndrome
MMC	myelomeningocele
NET	neuroendocrine tumor
NPARM	non-polyalanine repeat mutation
NPV	negative pressure ventilation
OSA	obstructive sleep apnea
PAP	positive airway pressure
PARM	polyalanine repeat mutation
PPV	positive pressure ventilation
PR	pulse rate
PSG	polysomnogram
PWS	Prader–Willi syndrome
REM	rapid eye movement
ROHHAD	rapid-onset obesity with hypothalamic dysfunction, hypoventilation and autonomic dysregulation
SDB	sleep disordered breathing
$TcCO_2$	transcutaneous carbon dioxide
TST	total sleep time

under 1 year of age may include a decrease in heart rate to less than 50 beats/min for at least 5 seconds or less than 60 beats/min for 15 seconds.[3] An event is scored as a central hypopnea if *none* of the following criteria are met: (1) snoring during the event, (2) increased inspiratory flattening of the nasal pressure or positive airway pressure (PAP) device flow signal compared with baseline breathing, and (3) an associated thoracoabdominal paradox occurs during the event but not during the pre-event breathing. Periodic breathing is defined as $\geq$3 episodes of central apnea lasting greater than 3 seconds each, and separated by $\leq$ 20 seconds of normal breathing.[3] Periodic breathing occurs relatively frequently in premature infants or children at high altitude and is occasionally seen in older children with central nervous system abnormalities, or as a brief normal phenomenon at sleep onset.

The International Classification of Sleep Disorders (ICSD)-3 recognizes 6 different forms of CSA, including primary CSA, and CSA due to other causes such as Cheyne-Stokes breathing, medical conditions, drugs or substances, high altitude periodic breathing, and infancy.[1] In the pediatric population beyond infancy (infancy being a time period wherein breathing is characterized by central apneas and periodic breathing), CSA occurs more commonly in association with underlying medical conditions, as outlined in **Box 1**.[4] CSA can also occur in the context of other sleep-disordered breathing conditions such as OSA, congenital central hypoventilation syndrome (CCHS), rapid-onset obesity with hypothalamic dysfunction, hypoventilation and autonomic dysregulation (ROHHAD), Prader-Willi syndrome (PWS), Leigh syndrome (LS), Chiari malformation (CM), brain tumors, neuromuscular disorders, and may also emerge with treatment.[5]

Diagnosis of Pediatric Central Sleep Apnea

A full-night in-laboratory PSG is the gold standard diagnostic test to diagnose CSA.[3] However, the minimum number of central events associated with a disease or a specific disorder or syndrome remains elusive and may be different between patient populations. As such, there is no defined and validated threshold for the number of central apneas associated with the disease. Normative data in healthy children have observed that short duration (<20 seconds) of central apneas during sleep are considered physiologic, particularly in the context of sigh, movement, and/or rapid eye movement (REM) sleep.[5] There is an age-related decrease in central apneas that is thought to be related to the maturation of the central nervous system.[6,7] Frequency of central apneas at 1 year of age was reviewed in a birth cohort study of 562 healthy infants who had PSG data obtained in their home settings at a mean age of 1.1$\pm$0.2 years. Central apneas, which were scored according to AASM criteria, were uncommon, with a median CAI of 2.5 events per hour (10th percentile 0.6, 90th percentile 7.0 events per hour).[8] In older, healthy children 3 to 7 years of age, a CAI greater than 1/h was uncommon and rarely associated with significant oxygen desaturations and/or arousal.[9] Data from several studies suggest that nonphysiological CSA should be suspected when the CAI is greater than 5 events per hour. This is particularly true when apneas are frequently associated with significant oxygen desaturations, occur in both non-REM (NREM) sleep and REM sleep, and each lasts longer than 10 seconds.[4,5] More recent data also suggest a higher CAI of around 10 events per hour is more likely to be associated with structural MRI abnormalities.[10] It is important to note that these parameters may not apply to healthy infants

Box 1
Pediatric classification of central sleep apnea

Physiologic

- Sleep onset
- Post-arousal
- Post-sigh breath
- Phasic REM sleep
- Body movement
- Sleep-wake transition
- High altitude

CSA with Genetic Conditions

- CCHS
- Down syndrome
- Prader–Willi syndrome
- Rett syndrome
- Vici syndrome
- Joubert syndrome
- Smith-Magenis syndrome
- Achondroplasia

CSA with Neurologic Disorder

- Arnold-Chiari malformation
- Central nervous system tumors
- Absence of corpus callosum
- Neuromuscular diseases
- Epilepsy

CSA with Cardiac Diseases

- Idiopathic pulmonary hypertension
- Cardiomyopathy
- Heart failure
- Tetralogy of Fallot

CSA with Thoracic and Primary Abnormalities

- Laryngomalacia
- Choanal atresia
- Thoracic cage abnormalities

CSA Related to Medications

- Opioids
- Baclofen
- Sodium oxybate

CSA Related to Lung Diseases

- Bronchopulmonary dysplasia

CSA Related to Congenital Craniofacial Disorders

- Craniosynostosis
- Pierre-Robin sequence

CSA with Infections

- RSV bronchiolitis
- Meningitis
- Encephalitis

CSA in Other Conditions

- Inborn errors of metabolism
- Gastro-esophageal reflux
- Chronic renal failure and patients on dialysis
- Traumatic brain injury

CSA with Endocrine Abnormalities

- ROHHAD syndrome
- Obesity
- Hypothyroidism

CSA Co-existing with SDB and SDB Treatments

- Obstructive sleep apnea
- CPAP emergent CSA
- HFNC emergent CSA

Abbreviations: CCHS, congenital central hypoventilation syndrome; CPAP, continuous positive airway pressure; CSA, central sleep apnea; HFNC, high flow nasal cannula; REM, rapid eye movement; ROHHAD, rapid-onset obesity with hypothalamic dysfunction, hypoventilation, and autonomic dysregulation; RSV, respiratory syncytial virus; SDB, sleep disordered breathing.

and children who reside at high altitude (2640 m) where the median (5th–95th centile) CAI in infants less than 45 days, 3 to 4 months, 6 to 7 months, and 10 to 18 months, were 12.4 (2.2–65.4), 8.3 (1.6–50.7), 5.5 (0.8–17.8), and 2.3 (0.7–8.7) events per hour respectively, with nadir SaO_2 levels during respiratory events being 70%, 72%, 76%, and 80%, respectively.[11]

Prevalence

Based on the criteria of CAI greater than 5 events per hour in non-preterm babies and children, 25/969 (2.5%) met the criteria for CSA in one unselected retrospective cohort study of both healthy children and children with underlying medical complexity.[4] However, using the same criteria, CSA prevalence has been reported to be significantly higher in other groups; 43% in infants with laryngomalacia,[12] 50% in infants with PWS,[13] and 60% in children diagnosed with Arnold CM.[14]

Clinical Manifestations

The clinical presentation of CSA can vary from an incidental finding in an asymptomatic child with a history of restless sleep to frank apneas and hypersomnolence in others.[4,15] Many children with a PSG diagnosis of CSA have been found to be asymptomatic, such as those with chronic kidney disease, Arnold–Chiari malformations, achondroplasia, and Down syndrome.[4,15,16] On the contrary, some children may present with symptoms related to sleep-related breathing disorders, specifically OSA symptoms such as snoring, with CSA being an incidental finding or coexisting with OSA, for example, in children with Arnold–Chiari malformation.[17] The presence of CSA may also predict the prognosis of a disease. For instance, CSA in infants with congenital heart disease is associated with a 4-fold increase in mortality.[18]

Evaluation and Management of Pediatric Central Sleep Apnea

Investigations should be directed by the clinical examination, the PSG findings, and the underlying etiology of CSA (**Box 2**). The management of CSA must be targeted toward its underlying cause and severity, particularly in the presence of oxygen desaturations and hypercapnia. Therapeutics and management may include oxygen, acetazolamide, noninvasive positive pressure ventilation (PPV), or caffeine. Some reports also cite the beneficial effects of melatonin through the stabilization of sleep.[5,19] Although caffeine has been historically used for AOP, there are data to suggest that infants at 36 weeks of gestation treated with caffeine had a significantly reduced frequency of central apneas, possibly through the increased frequency of arousals to hypoxic episodes.[20] Two retrospective studies on infants with CSA indicate a generally positive clinical outcome in early life. The first study of 18 infants showed that treatments such as supplemental oxygen, caffeine, and noninvasive ventilation led to significant improvements over 12 months, and 60% of them discontinued respiratory support at a median (interquartile range [IQR]) age of 1.02 (0.93–1.04) years.[21] The second study suggested that CSA in healthy term infants under 1 year old also has a good prognosis, with a duration of supplemental oxygen therapy for a median of 6 months, resulting in improved oxygen saturation and reduced apnea-hypopnea index.[22] Ultimately, with the trajectory of CSA remaining unclear, a conservative monitoring approach using oxygen saturation monitoring and/or PSG surveillance may be the management of choice in some children.

Box 2
Evaluation for central sleep apnea

- Complete neurologic evaluation
- MRI Brain ± MRI C-spine
- EEG
- Brainstem evoked potentials
- Genetic panels—CCHS, PWS
- ECG
- Echocardiogram
- Thyroid function tests
- Chest X ray
- Urine electrolytes and toxicology
- Flexible nasolaryngoscopy
- Evaluation for gastro-esophageal reflux

Abbreviations: ECG, electrocardiogram; EEG, electroencephalogram; CCHS, congenital central hypoventilation syndrome; PWS, Prader-Willi syndrome.

Summary

CSA in children cannot be reliably identified or diagnosed on the basis of history alone as there are no discrete set of signs and/or symptoms and a PSG is required to confirm a diagnosis. A high index of suspicion and referral for PSG or the need for regular surveillance with PSGs must be considered in the context of a specific underlying disorder. Moreover, although CSA is relatively uncommon in childhood, it is likely underdiagnosed due to a lack of distinct symptomology. Finally, it would be important to understand the natural course of CSA from childhood to adulthood and to identify the long-term outcomes of children with CSA.

CENTRAL HYPOVENTILATION DISORDERS

Introduction

Central hypoventilation (CH) disorders in children include a spectrum of disorders in which respiratory insufficiency results from abnormalities of central respiratory control. Both congenital and secondary CH disorders can have anatomic and/or functional abnormalities resulting in disordered respiratory control. These abnormalities may occur at the level of controllers (brain and brainstem), sensors (central and peripheral chemoreceptors), or along signaling pathways between controllers, sensors, and ventilatory muscles.

Definitions and Terminology

The definitions of hypoventilation, based on P_{CO_2} values, apply to both obstructive and central disorders and are not pediatric-specific. A daytime (awake) P_{CO_2} greater than 45 mm Hg is generally considered helpful for the diagnosis of hypoventilation in both adults and children.[23] Nocturnal hypoventilation is, however, more accurately characterized during an overnight polysomnogram (PSG). In children, the AASM defines nocturnal hypoventilation on a PSG as P_{CO_2} (as measured by end-tidal or transcutaneous capnography) greater than 50 mm Hg for at least 25% of total sleep time (TST).[3,24] For children greater than 13 years of age and adults, other commonly applied definitions of hypoventilation include P_{CO_2} greater than 55 mm Hg for $\geq$10 minutes, or an increase in P_{CO_2} greater than 10 mm Hg above awake supine readings if sleep values reach greater than 50 mm Hg for at least 10 minutes.[2] Ventilation varies by sleep stage due to dynamic changes in both ventilatory muscle function and respiratory control. The transition from wakefulness to initial stages of NREM results in a decrease in muscle tone and overall decreases in minute ventilation, resulting in an increase in P_{CO_2} and a decrease in SaO_2. When accounting for variability across all sleep stages, P_{CO_2} can increase to 6 mm Hg above awake baseline across the night and the average SaO_2 are 1% to 2% lower than awake baseline.[25]

CONGENITAL CENTRAL HYPOVENTILATION SYNDROME

Introduction

CCHS is a rare disorder of the autonomic nervous system (ANS) characterized by absent ventilatory responses to hypoxia and hypercapnia. CCHS is a global dysautonomia,[26] with abnormalities that adversely affect multiple systems in addition to CH.[27] An estimated 3000 to 5000 individuals with CCHS are identified worldwide, with an estimated prevalence of 1/100,000 to 1/500,000.[27,28]

Genetics and Diagnosis

CCHS is caused by mutations of the paired-like homeobox (*PHOX2b*) gene on chromosome 4p12, which is critical for the development of the ANS. Approximately 90% of cases are caused by heterozygote polyalanine repeat mutations (PARMs) with 24 to 33 repeat sequences (normal genotypes carry 20 repeat sequences on both copies).[27] Non-PARM (NPARM) mutations account for approximately 10% of those with CCHS, including frameshift, missense, nonsense, stop codons, and splice-site mutations. Rare partial and whole gene deletions/duplications have also been reported.[27,29–32] Recommended sequential testing for *PHOX2b* includes fragment analysis screening, gene sequencing, and rarely, gene-specific deletion/duplication analysis (**Table 1**). The vast majority including those with asymptomatic mosaic abnormalities are found on screening or sequencing.[27] Most cases are due to *de novo* mutations, but autosomal dominant transmission is also well documented.[33,34]

Clinical Manifestations

The primary finding is hypoventilation in the absence of other respiratory, cardiac, neurologic, or metabolic abnormalities. Ventilatory responses to hypoxia and hypercapnia are absent or severely diminished, most pronounced while asleep, more variably while awake. In a sleep study, hypoventilation is worse in NREM sleep compared with REM sleep, which is not typical of other CH disorders (see **Table 1**).[35] Respiratory rates tend to be monotonous with shallow volumes. Nonrespiratory dysautonomias, discussion of which is beyond the scope of this review, are common and often can be more complicated to treat than CH. Neurobehavioral and cognitive function are wide-ranging, with neurodiverse conditions common.[36]

Onset can occur in the neonatal period or late-onset after 1 month of age (see **Table 1**).[27,28,37] Neonatal presentation can include respiratory arrest at birth, intermittent hypoxemia particularly with sleeping and feeding, severe breath-holding spells, and/or central apneas, sometimes misclassified as periodic breathing, and all can result in respiratory failure.[38] Respiratory distress such as tachypnea is not present. Late-onset CCHS is less common and occurs after the first month of life.[28,37] Affected individuals phenotypically tend to be less severe, even asymptomatic, but abnormal ventilatory patterns are similar to neonatal-onset CCHS.[28,37] Hypoventilation may be uncovered with acute illness, anesthesia, opioids, sleep studies obtained for other clinical indications, or genetic testing of parents of children with confirmed CCHS.[37,39]

Genotype/phenotype correlations have been made. Among those with PARMs, individuals with longer PARMs (20/27–20/33) tend to have more severe hypoventilation including needing more ventilatory support during wakefulness,[27,28] cardiac arrythmias requiring pacemaker placement,[40] Hirschsprung's or chronic constipation,[41] higher likelihood for neural crest tumors (though overall still relatively rare in PARMs)[27] and possibly more impaired neurocognitive function.[42] Severity of hypoventilation in those with NPARMs varies widely.[43–46] Hirschsprung's disease and neural crest tumors occur in up to 80% to 100% and 50% to 60% of NPARM cases, respectively.[47] Patterns between neurocognitive function and

Table 1
Respiratory disturbance and management plan for children with CCHS, ROHHAD, and PWS

Diagnosis	Typical Respiratory Disturbance Features and Symptoms	Diagnostic Methods	Management Plan for Respiratory Disturbance
CCHS	Primarily hypoventilation • Absent or diminished ventilatory responses to hypoxia and hypercapnia • Worse during sleep compared with wake • Worse in non-REM sleep and better in REM sleep Neonatal onset (within 1-mo of age) • Respiratory arrest at birth • Intermittent hypoxemia particularly with sleeping and feeding • Severe breath holding spells • Central apneas sometimes misclassified as periodic breathing • Respiratory failure Late-onset (after 1-mo of age) • Similar ventilatory patterns to neonatal-onset CCHS • Less severe, even asymptomatic	Testing for *PHOX2b* mutation • Fragment analysis screening • Gene sequencing • Gene specific deletion/ duplication analysis	• Positive pressure ventilation (PPV) via tracheostomy or mask • Negative pressure ventilation • Diaphragm pacing (DP) via phrenic nerve stimulation
ROHHAD	• Hypoventilation ○ Usually nocturnal but it can occur during daytime as well ○ Not evident at disease onset ○ Present after weight gain and hypothalamic dysfunction • Central sleep apnea • Obstructive sleep apnea • Daytime hypoventilation	Based on clinical sign and symptoms (see **Box 3**)	See **Table 2**
PWS	• Hypoventilation • OSA • CSA • Reduced response to hypoxia and hypercapnia • Decreased pulmonary function	Based on genetic testing	• Low flow O2 (usually weaned off by 2 y of age) • Noninvasive ventilation is needed if unresponsive to O2

genotypes have not been clearly established in NPARM individuals.[42,48]

Ventilatory Management of Congenital Central Hypoventilation Syndrome

Nearly all individuals with CCHS have lifelong dependence on assisted ventilation during sleep, with variable needs during the day. Optimal ventilation should maintain SaO_2 greater than 95% and Pco_2 between 35 to 45 mm Hg, while minimizing atelectasis and barotrauma.[28,43] Elective hyperventilation to Pco_2 between 30 and 35 mm Hg may increase the length of daytime sprinting off support.[49] Supplemental oxygen is typically not needed.[28] Settings are best titrated noninvasively during sleep at routine intervals, but must provide guaranteed respiratory rates and guaranteed inspiratory times. Supplemental oxygen alone is not sufficient treatment and may actually worsen hypoventilation.[50] Use of pharmacologic agents to treat CCHS is not reliably effective and hence not suggested as monotherapy.[28,51,52]

Objective monitoring with continuous overnight oximetry and appropriate ventilator-enabled alarms with ranges set to avoid frequent nuisance alarms is crucial in CCHS management.[28] Capnography is ideal but difficult to obtain, and it becomes even more challenging with mask ventilation. Those with CCHS arouse less frequently to standard alarms, further iterating the need for trained health care workers overnight.[53]

Increase of ventilatory support may be needed during sedentary behavior, illnesses, and/or with exercise, particularly in more severe genotypes.[54] Support should be augmented when undergoing any sedation/anesthesia for procedures, especially at induction.[54]

There are 4 major modalities of ventilatory assistance: (1) PPV via tracheostomy, (2) PPV via mask, (3) negative pressure ventilation (NPV), or (4) diaphragm pacing (DP) via phrenic nerve stimulation (see **Table 1**). At times, combinations of these modalities are needed to maintain support during sleep and wake.

1. PPV via tracheostomy is the most robust and guaranteed delivery system but also the most invasive. If used, most can be supported with an uncuffed tracheostomy tube using a pressure-limited modality with timed rate and guaranteed inspiratory time, set to age-typical ranges. Newer mixed ventilation modes are available if desired.[55]
2. PPV via mask is delivered via a bi-level PAP machine or home ventilator, the latter of which is preferred given more alarms and portability.[28,56] Full-face masks are preferred to minimize oral leak and mid-face pressure. Mask use for greater than 16 h/d is not recommended given mask interference with daily activities, impairment of social and physical development, and potential mid-face hypoplasia.[57,58] The use of PPV-mask in infants is challenging but not impossible and requires consideration of infants' longer TSTs, frequent and unpredictable sleep-wake transitions, and less stable pulmonary mechanics.[58] Careful monitoring for midface retrusion is recommended.[59] Transitioning to mask ventilation can allow for tracheostomy decannulation.[60,61] Suggested protocols for decannulation and transition to mask ventilation are reviewed elsewhere.[60,61] Should decannulation be desired for an individual requiring 24 h/d ventilatory support, the use of nocturnal PPV via mask and DP while awake is possible.
3. NPV can be delivered via chest wall interface (e.g., cuirass) but is not portable, and rarely used in CCHS. Challenges include leak and airway occlusion with NPV breaths.[28,62,63]
4. Diaphragm pacing (DP) via phrenic nerve stimulation results in diaphragmatic contraction and subsequent negative inspiration. Details of DP placement and use are reviewed elsewhere.[64,65] A phrenic nerve stimulator system is FDA-approved for those with CCHS which is small and portable; however, it should not be confused with intramuscular diaphragm pacing systems.[66] DP is best when used less than 12 to 16 h/d, either during sleep alone or during wake with PPV during sleep.[64] Safe, long-term use has been described in adults up to 40 years after placement, including in pregnancy.[33,67] Cardiac pacemakers and vagal nerve stimulators can be used with DP.[67,68] Challenges include (1) additional surgeries for routine replacement of parts or complications,[69] (2) limited alarms signaling malfunction of leads or transmitter, (3) MRI incompatibility, (4) possible upper airway obstruction with paced breaths which cannot be predicted and may preclude tracheostomy decannulation,[60,61,70–73] (5) lack of automatic use, that is, transmitter needs to be manually turned on/off with each use, is battery-operated, antennae (not wireless) need to be manually placed over receivers daily, and (6) PPV-mask ventilation must be available and tolerated in case of DP failure.

Discussion

Future directions in CCHS include further research around molecular understanding of *PHOX2b*'s pathogenic role in CCHS, with the hope of developing a cure or treatment beyond current supportive measures, improving in home monitoring and ventilatory modalities, expanding the understanding of genotype/phenotype correlations, and learning more about adults with CCHS.

Summary

CCHS is a rare disorder caused by abnormalities of *PHOX2b* leading to diminished ventilatory and arousal responses to hypoxia and hypercapnia, lifelong dependence on ventilatory assistance during sleep and variably during wake, and other nonrespiratory dysautonomias. There is no known cure, and life expectancy is unknown. There is emerging data linking more severe phenotypes that have worsened hypoventilation and more dysautonomias to more severe genotypes. Common ventilatory management options include PPV-tracheostomy, PPV-mask, and DP. Importantly, comprehensive and collaborative treatment of CCHS includes the nonrespiratory dysautonomias, many of which can be more challenging to treat than the hypoventilation.

RAPID-ONSET OBESITY WITH HYPOTHALAMIC DYSFUNCTION, HYPOVENTILATION, AND AUTONOMIC DYSREGULATION SYNDROME

Background

ROHHAD is a rare disease first described by Fishman and colleagues in 1965.[74] It is a heterogeneous syndrome, characterized by a variable presentation and a constellation of symptoms.[75] Over the past 60 years, approximately 200 cases of ROHHAD have been reported worldwide.[76–80] However, it is highly probable that numerous patients suffering from this condition remain undiagnosed. Notably, its distinct clinical phenotype differentiates it from other overlapping complex disorders, such as Prader-Willi Disease or CCHS. This includes a relative absence of symptoms at birth, a lack of known genetic abnormalities, and is dominated by the sudden onset of weight gain with associated hyperphagia among previously healthy pre-school-aged children.

Clinical Manifestations

The diagnosis of ROHHAD is challenging as no genetic basis or pathognomonic biomarker has been identified.[75,81,82] Currently, ROHHAD is diagnosed based on clinical criteria and recognizing the clinical manifestations of ROHHAD is critical for the prompt diagnosis and management of this disorder. Disease onset begins in early childhood, typically between 2 and 4 years of age (2–15 years age range reported in childhood) with data suggesting a female-to-male ratio of 2:1.[76] The clinical diagnostic criteria for ROHHAD include the presence of (1) rapid-onset obesity, (2) hypothalamic dysfunction, (3) hypoventilation, and (4) autonomic dysregulation. More recently, the recognition of the association of ROHHAD syndrome with neuroendocrine tumors (NETs) has been included in the acronym, ROHHADNET.[80] In aggregate patient data of a total of 110 pediatric patients, rapid onset obesity was observed in 65% of children, hypoventilation in 46%, hypothalamic dysfunction in 78%, and autonomic dysfunction in 75% with behavioral changes in 36%.[77] Neuroendocrine tumors were reported in 42% of patients with ganglioneuroma being the most common. The clinical symptoms and manifestations of ROHHAD impact many systems of the body and are variable in their presence, severity, and timing such that they may evolve, fluctuate, and/or stabilize over time which hinders both the diagnosis and management of the condition.[75,78,83] Specific abnormalities are highlighted below underscoring the importance of understanding the variability of ROHHAD.

Rapid onset obesity

The most common symptom at disease onset is hyperphagia and rapid weight gain leading to obesity. Typically, the weight gain is significant with an increase of 20 to 40 pounds over 6 to 12 months.[75,84] Prior to this, children with ROHHAD syndrome usually have normal growth and development.[75,84]

Hypothalamic dysfunction

Evidence for pituitary hormone dysfunction may present months to years following the rapid increase in weight.[75] Hypothalamic changes include growth hormone (GH) deficiency, central hypothyroidism, diabetes insipidus, syndrome of inappropriate anti-diuretic hormone, adrenal insufficiency, hyperprolactinemia, as well as precocious or delayed puberty.[75,76,81–85] Common laboratory findings include dysnatremia (hypernatremia and, less commonly, hyponatremia), hyperprolactinemia, decreased insulin growth factor-1 (IGF-1) levels, and hypothyroidism.[76,77]

Hypoventilation, respiratory, and sleep disorders

Nocturnal hypoventilation, specifically nocturnal hypercapnia as per AASM criteria is considered to be central to the diagnosis of ROHHAD and often co-exists with central apneas at night as well during wakefulness.[3] However, hypoventilation may not be evident at disease onset and indeed may not be present until further into the course of the disease after the dramatic weight gain and hypothalamic dysfunction,[86] which may result in the misclassification of a patient as simple obesity and delay a clinical diagnosis of ROHHAD. Other respiratory and sleep-related abnormalities also may co-exist and include obstructive sleep apnea (OSA), CSA, narcolepsy, and/or sleep disturbance as well as daytime hypoventilation, bradypnea, and hypoxia (see **Table 1**).[76,83,87]

Respiratory instability Children with ROHHAD syndrome may initially present with acute hypercapnic respiratory failure following a minor respiratory illness or anesthesia requiring intubation and ventilation.[76,77,79,83,88,89] In one study consisting of 15 children with ROHHAD, all with a diagnosis of nocturnal hypoventilation, 9/15 had experienced a cardiorespiratory arrest and 4/9 displayed evidence of respiratory instability from 2 months to a few days prior to the arrest.[75] Respiratory instability was characterized as oxygen desaturations during sleep, cyanotic episodes, and OSA. In contrast, hypoventilation may not always be evident at the initial presentation. In a retrospective cohort study of 6 children with ROHHAD syndrome, Reppucci and colleagues observed that the median age of rapid-onset obesity was 3.5 years and at presentation, only 2/6 children had nocturnal hypoventilation on a baseline PSG while the remaining 4/6 had OSA only. PSG surveillance every 6 to 12 months was continued in this cohort and the remaining 4/6 children showed the evolution of respiratory instability with progression to nocturnal hypoventilation at a median age of 7.5 years,[83] highlighting that OSA may be an important early finding in children with suspected ROHHAD syndrome.[75,83] Other markers of respiratory instability may be evident on both an overnight PSG and during daytime (awake) cardiorespiratory monitoring. In a study of 8 children with ROHHAD along with 8 sex and BMI matched controls who did not have nocturnal hypoventilation, there were no significant differences in the overall obstructive apnea-hypopnea index (OAHI, 11.1 vs 12.1 events per hour, respectively), central apnea index (CAI, 0.1 vs 0.5 events per hour, respectively) or nadir SaO_2 (80.2 vs 82.0%, respectively) as observed on overnight PSG. However, children with ROHHAD had a significantly higher desaturation index compared with controls (37.9/h vs 14.7/h, respectively). Of note, the high desaturation index in children with ROHHAD was out of keeping with the observed number of obstructive and/or central events.[88] Moreover, daytime cardiorespiratory monitoring during quiet wakefulness, which was performed in a standardized manner over 4 hours the morning after PSG monitoring, demonstrated the presence of central apneas with associated mild to severe oxygen desaturations (**Fig. 1**).[88]

Furthermore, there is increasing recognition of children with ROHHAD presenting with excessive daytime sleepiness consistent with narcolepsy and cataplexy, with evidence of decreased hypocretin levels in cerebrospinal fluid.[87] Screening for narcolepsy through questionnaires and monitoring with a multiple sleep latency test should be considered for every child with ROHHAD where there are concerns for excessive daytime sleepiness and suspected narcolepsy.

Etiology of respiratory instability The cause of ventilatory abnormalities observed in ROHHAD is not well elucidated. Overall, the breathing abnormalities observed are believed to be due to abnormal or blunted ventilatory responses to hypoxia and hypercapnia, both during sleep and wakefulness.[90] Blunted chemosensory responses may be associated with dysregulation of the orexinergic system, as indicated by reduced or absent levels of cerebrospinal orexin (also called hypocretin) in children with ROHHAD.[82,87] Orexinergic neurons, which contribute to a state of wakefulness, are recognized as central chemoreceptors that facilitate and mediate cardiorespiratory responses in response to high carbon dioxide levels, resulting in a hypercapnic ventilatory reflex.[91] Additionally, respiratory abnormalities observed during rest while awake may be a result of diminished tidal volumes and inspiratory drive. However, limited data suggest that submaximal exercise does not exacerbate respiratory instability.[88] This is due to increases in tidal volume resulting from physical activity triggered by the activation of central thermoreceptors and mechanoreceptors in the muscles and joints.[92,93] Finally, it has been reported that one of the major effects of hypothyroidism is its influence on central ventilatory control and that both hypoxic and hypercapnic ventilatory impairments are significantly present in untreated hypothyroidism, as observed in ROHHAD syndrome.[92–95]

Autonomic dysregulation

A wide spectrum of autonomic abnormalities has been observed in ROHHAD syndrome which includes dysautonomic features such as altered perception of pain, temperature dysregulation, arrhythmias, abnormal heart rate such as tachycardia or bradycardia, and alterations in blood pressure with either hypertension or hypotension,[77–79] gastrointestinal dysmotility,[79] and ophthalmologic abnormalities such as blurred vision, strabismus, and atypical pupillary responses to light.[76]

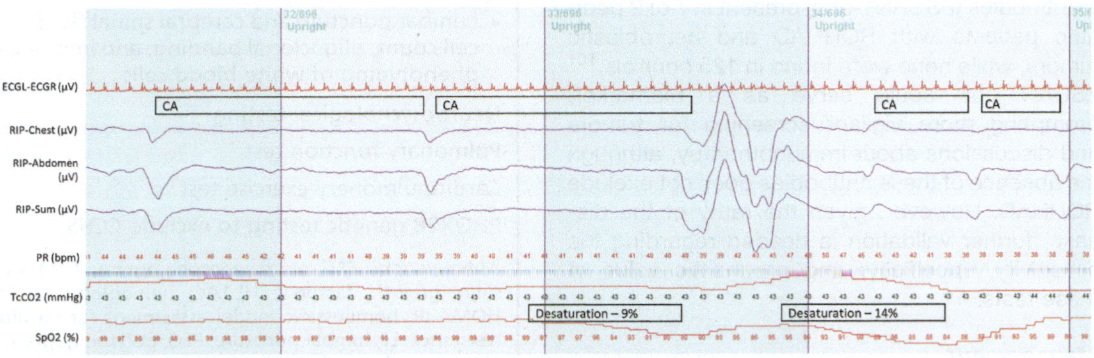

Fig. 1. Cardiopulmonary monitoring during wakefulness in a child with ROHHAD syndrome. Note-evidence of central apneas associated with oxygen desaturations while awake. CA, central apnea; PR, pulse rate; $TcCO_2$, transcutaneous carbon dioxide.

Neuroendocrine tumors

Neuroendocrine tumors (NETs) arise from cells that originate in the neural crest, and some authors have adopted the acronym ROHHAD (NET) to account for their presence. In 2 systematic reviews of collated data with sample sizes of 43 and 110 children, respectively (the studies likely include many of the same children), approximately 40% to 56% of the patients with ROHHAD syndrome developed tumors of neural crest origin, commonly ganglioneuromas and less often ganglioneuroblastomas.[76,77] These tumors were localized in the abdomen, chest, or along the sympathetic nervous system chain, with the majority in the adrenal area with 2 reported cases of mediastinal masses,[77] highlighting the need for ongoing surveillance.

Diagnosis

There are no single genetic or pathognomonic biomarkers currently available, and the evaluation and diagnosis are based on clinical signs and symptoms (**Box 3**).[74,75,83,84] In one study, whole-exome sequencing was utilized to analyze 35 ROHHAD children including an unaffected monozygotic twin (with another twin displaying classic ROHHAD phenotype) and tumors (ganglioneuromas and ganglioneuroblastomas in chest or abdomen) from 4 children with ROHHAD,[96,97] but there were no identified pathogenetic mutations and/or structural variations in the exomes, suggesting that whole-exome sequencing may not be a useful diagnostic test for ROHHAD syndrome.[98,99] Autoimmune-mediated processes have also been illustrated by the variable beneficial impact of intensive immunosuppressive treatment on symptoms, respiratory manifestations, and neuropsychological function.[100]

More recently, Zinc finger and SCAN domain-containing protein 1 (ZSCAN1) has been identified as a candidate autoantigen in ROHHAD, with autoantibodies (ZSCAN1-abs) present in 7 of 9 pediatric patients with ROHHAD and neuroblastic tumors, while none were found in 125 controls.[101] ZSCAN1-abs could serve as a biomarker, prompting more vigilant screening for tumors and discussions about immunotherapy, although the absence of these antibodies does not exclude ROHHAD. However, given the rarity of the disease, further validation is needed regarding the sensitivity, specificity, and prognostic value of these tests.

Box 3
Evaluation for rapid-onset obesity with hypothalamic dysfunction, hypoventilation, and autonomic dysregulation syndrome

Anthropometrics to evaluate trajectory of height, weight, BMI, and Tanner stage

Temperature

Hypothalamic function

- Prolactin, TSH, free T4, IGF-1, luteinizing hormone, follicle stimulating hormone, estradiol or testosterone, cortisol, 24-h cortisol urine test

Metabolic function

- Fasting blood glucose, HOMA-IR, HbA1c, lipid profile, liver enzymes
- Serum electrolytes and complete blood count
- Urine electrolytes, urine osmolarity
- Urine spot homovanillic acid, vanillylmandelic acid, norepinephrine, epinephrine, dopamine, metanephrine

Autonomic/Cardiovascular

- 24-h ambulatory blood pressure
- Echocardiogram
- Holter (24 h minimum)
- Ophthalmology assessment
- Cardiopulmonary exercise test

Hypoventilation

- Overnight level 1 PSG
- Daytime monitoring with PSG during quiet wakefulness

Neural Crest Tumor Screen/Evaluation

- MRI of brain/brainstem/chest/abdomen
- Ultrasound abdomen

Neurologic

- Electroencephalogram
- Lumbar puncture and cerebral spinal fluid for cell count, oligoclonal banding, and immunophenotyping of white blood cells

Neuropsychological testing

Pulmonary function test

Cardiopulmonary exercise test

PHOX2B genetic testing to exclude CCHS

Abbreviations: EEG, electroencephalogram; IGF-1, insulin growth factor-1; Hb1Ac, hemoglobin A1C; HOMA-IR, homeostatic model assessment for insulin resistance; LP, lumbar puncture; PSG, polysomnogram; TSH, thyroid stimulating hormone.

Management

The broad management (**Table 2**) of children with ROHHAD syndrome requires a coordinated and

Table 2
Management approaches for ROHHAD syndrome

Clinical Manifestations	Management Approaches
Weight gain	• Diet • Physical activity program • Bariatric surgery
Hypothalamic dysfunction Hypothyroidism Hyperprolactinemia Growth hormone deficiency Adrenal insufficiency Pubertal delay Diabetes insipidus	• Specific hormone replacement
Respiratory instability and/or Hypoventilation Narcolepsy	• Nocturnal CPAP/bi-level PAP with or without supplemental oxygen • Tracheostomy and invasive ventilation during sleep or for 24 h during wakefulness and sleep • Diaphragm pacing • Daytime supplemental oxygen • Stimulant medication for narcolepsy
Autonomic dysregulation Cardiovascular Gastrointestinal Neuropsychological Thermal	• Antihypertensive medication • Cardiac pacemaker • Stool softener • Anti-epileptics • Antidepressants and antianxiety medication • Regulation of ambient temperature
Metabolic disorders	• Diuretics • Electrolyte replacement • Regulate glucose • Antidiabetic drugs • Lipid lowering agents
Neural crest tumors	• Surgical removal • Conservative—watch-and-wait

Abbreviation: CPAP, continuous positive airway pressure.

collaborative inter-professional care approach which is critical in minimizing long-term morbidity. Given the rarity and complexity of the disease as well as the clinical variability and course of ROHHAD, it is evident that there are no standardized therapeutic approaches for the management of ROHHAD, emphasizing the need for individualized treatment which must be optimized for every child on a regular basis.

Ventilatory management

All children with ROHHAD with evidence of nocturnal hypoventilation will require either nocturnal ventilatory support with non-invasive ventilation such as bi-level PAP, or invasive ventilation via a tracheostomy which may be required either solely during sleep or in more severe cases, for 24 hours a day. Additionally, many of these children may require supplemental oxygen during the day and/or night with prescribed ventilatory support, especially in those with evidence of intermittent hypoxia on daytime oximetry and/or pulmonary hypertension.[88,102] Early intervention with nocturnal noninvasive or invasive ventilation has been suggested to improve ventilation during both sleep and wakefulness.[103] Children maintained on ventilatory support should have, at a minimum, yearly evaluations of their control of breathing during wakefulness and sleep with PSG monitoring, although these may be required earlier if there is a concern for respiratory instability despite using nocturnal ventilation or a change in clinical manifestations.

For children without evidence of nocturnal hypoventilation or other symptoms of sleep-disordered breathing at presentation, but with a strong suspicion for ROHHAD, close and serial monitoring with PSGs every 6 to 12 months where available, including daytime monitoring of cardiopulmonary variables, is recommended.[83] It is important to note that some children, with or without respiratory support who appeared to be clinically stable, can present with acute respiratory failure requiring intubation and ventilation.[77]

Long-term Outcomes and Prognosis

The long-term outcomes and prognoses for children diagnosed with ROHHAD are not well understood. In addition to the high degree of multiple morbidities, there is a high risk of mortality in childhood. One dataset reported 12 deaths in an aggregated set of 110 children. Of these, 9 of 12 were due to sudden cardiorespiratory arrest, although more specific data on the exact cause of death and data on the remaining 3 children were not provided.[76] There are several cases of children with ROHHAD surviving into adolescence and adulthood albeit with limited data on their clinical outcomes.[78,104] Novel clinical features not previously associated with ROHHAD have been identified, such as liver cirrhosis and hepatocellular carcinoma, suggesting that the disease continues to evolve beyond the pediatric years.[104]

PRADER–WILLI SYNDROME

Background

Prader–Willi syndrome (PWS) is a rare multisystem disorder affecting approximately 1 in 15,000 live births PWS derives from the loss of function of paternally expressed 15q11-q13 genes as a result of either a paternally derived de novo deletion of this region (61% of cases), maternal uniparental disomy of chromosome 15 (36%), or the silencing of the paternal alleles by an imprinting defect on the paternal chromosome (3%).[105–108]

Infants with PWS usually present with hypotonia, feeding difficulties and failure to thrive and a diagnosis is usually made with confirmatory genetic testing (see **Table 1**). In childhood and later in adult life, central nervous system and hypothalamic dysfunction are evidenced by hyperphagia leading to obesity after 2 to 4 years of age, temperature instability, sleep-disordered breathing, and multiple endocrine abnormalities, particularly GH deficiency.[105,109] In the last 2 decades, GH has become a mainstay of therapy for children with PWS and has been shown to increase adult height, neurocognitive function, exercise capacity, and body composition with increased muscle mass.[110,111]

Clinical Manifestations: Respiratory and Sleep Disorders

Hypoventilation, OSA, CSA, reduced response to hypoxia and hypercapnia, and decreased pulmonary function are more common in children with PWS than in the general population (see **Table 1**).[13,112–114] More specifically, data looking at PWS children (n = 44, median age 1.9 years), many of whom were GH naïve, noted the occurrence of CSA (defined as a CAI > 5/h), either isolated or co-existent with OSA, in 43% of the cohort and predominately in children less than 2 years of age.[113] However, OSA when present was mild in this age range. The frequency of central events correlated with younger age.[115] The frequency of CSA was uncommon beyond 2 years of age and rather OSA predominance was observed with a prevalence rate of 52% to 79%.[113] Of those with OSA, approximately 50% of children had mild OSA, and the remainder had moderate to severe OSA.[113,114] In a retrospective study including 16 obese children with PWS older than 2 years of age (median age = 11.5 years), 54.5% had a CAI exceeding 1/h, compared to 22.2% in the non-PWS control group.[116] However, all these studies defined CSA by CAI which does not account for central hypopneas. A case series including 17 children with a median (IQR) age of 11.6 (9.8–14.4) years showed that 8 out of 17 had CSA and their median (IQR) CAHI was 11.9 (8.2–20.0) events/hour, compared to the median (IQR) CAI of 1.9 (1.0–9.3) events/hour, suggesting that the majority of events were central hypopneas,[117] which highlights the possibility of underdiagnosis if central hypopneas are not included in the CSA definition.

Moreover, excessive daytime sleepiness and narcolepsy like symptoms have been reported in children with PWS that cannot be explained solely by the presence of OSA or night disturbances, with evidence for reduced CSF orexin levels in subjects with PWS.[118]

Pathophysiology

The etiology of CSA and OSA in PWS infants is thought to be multifactorial. Mechanisms contributing to CSA include hypotonia, brainstem immaturity, and hypothalamic dysfunction (such as central adrenal insufficiency[119]). Abnormal chemosensitivity to CO_2 and O_2, as well as altered arousal and cardiorespiratory responses to hypoxia, may cause respiratory depression.[112,120,121] The response to hypercapnia has been demonstrated to be further reduced in obese PWS children compared with non-obese PWS children and healthy, non-obese controls, although hypoxic ventilatory responses were absent or markedly reduced, independent of obesity in PWS.[121] Further studies demonstrate that these changes in ventilatory responses are modulated by primary peripheral chemoreceptor dysfunction and/or altered afferent pathways to central controllers.[49]

Management

The primary treatment strategy for CSA with associated oxygen desaturations is low-flow oxygen, with data to support that current treatment with supplemental oxygen not only improves oxygen saturation but also ameliorates central apneas (see **Table 1**).[113,122] As PWS subjects have abnormal chemosensitivity to both hypoxia and hypercapnia, even small degrees of hypoxia may likely have a destabilizing effect on the control of breathing, resulting in central depression, which is mitigated by low-flow oxygen. Usually, infants with PWS and co-existing CSA requiring oxygen are able to be weaned off oxygen by 2 years of age.[123] PWS infants with moderate to severe CSA who are unresponsive to oxygen may require noninvasive ventilation and, less rarely, invasive ventilation (see **Table 1**).[124] Until further conclusive evidence suggests otherwise, minimizing nocturnal oxygen desaturations and treating CSA should be considered in all infants with PWS.[113,122]

Children with PWS presenting with excessive daytime sleepiness should be screened with an MSLT and treated with stimulant medication such as methylphenidate or modafinil, as clinically indicated.[125,126] More recently, pitolisant, a histamine H3 receptor inverse agonist, improved daytime sleepiness as well as improvements in subjective cognition in children with PWS.[127]

OTHER HYPOVENTILATION DISORDERS

Introduction

Certain congenital or acquired CNS conditions can compromise central control of breathing, leading to wide-ranging sleep disordered breathing (SDB), including CSA, CH, and/or OSA. Abnormalities may be due to widespread neurologic dysfunctions or anatomic causes.

Anatomic Abnormalities

Generally, anatomic abnormalities in the posterior fossa and brainstem are thought to cause significant CH/CSA due to (postulated) disruption of respiratory control structures. Tumors in the brainstem, posterior fossa, and hypothalamic areas are associated with CSA, which can persist even into cancer survivorship.[128–133] CSA has recently been described in those with pontine tegmental cap dysplasia, and treatment of their CSA is complicated by contraindication to PPV-mask due to risk for severe corneal injuries.[134] A classic apnea-tachypnea pattern as well as CSA and OSA is seen in those with Joubert Syndrome, which is caused by agenesis/dysgenesis of the cerebellar vermis and diagnosed with the “molar tooth” sign on MRI.[135] Those with skeletal dysplasias, most commonly achondroplasia, frequently have OSA due to bony impact on the upper airway, but also have CSA thought to be related to brain stem dysfunction from cervico-occipital compression and foramen magnum stenosis.[136] Hypoventilation obviously is compounded by restrictive lung disease, and treatment for a spectrum of SDB in those with achondroplasia needs to be individualized.[136]

CMs are congenital hindbrain anomalies that can be categorized into 2 subtypes. CM type 1 (CM-I) involves downward herniation of the cerebellar tonsils, typically without myelomeningocele (MMC).[137] Respiratory control impairment and altered CO_2 sensitivity ensue, leading to periodic breathing and CSA.[138,139] Treatment involves surgical posterior fossa decompression, which may, but does not always improve CSA, and therefore supportive treatment for clinical respiratory insufficiency is required.[14,137,140] CM type II (CM-II) is characterized by herniation of the cerebellar vermis, caudal brain stem, and 4th ventricle through the foramen magnum, and is often associated with MMC, resulting in obstructive hydrocephalus. CSA, OSA, blunted ventilatory, and arousal responses to hypercapnia and hypoxia are present and can persist even after MMC repair.[141–143] Sudden death, possibly related to SDB, is known to occur in those with CM-II and MMC.[144]

Functional Abnormalities

Obesity hypoventilation syndrome (OHS) in children is diagnosed when body mass index greater than 95th percentile for age and sex, and hypercapnia during wakefulness (P_{CO_2} > 45 mm Hg) is present.[145] Prevalence is not well known, but likely underdiagnosed given the global obesity epidemic. Though most cases have concomitant OSA, not all do; hence, the role of central respiratory dysregulation as a phenotypic and endotypic variant of OSA, or as a stand-alone pathophysiologic pathway, warrants further exploration.[145]

LS is a genetic progressive neurodegenerative mitochondrial disease.[146,147] Both OSA and CSA have been described as well as a decreased arousal response to respiratory disturbances in sleep.[148] Common causes of death are respiratory insufficiency/failure or apneic events.[149]

Those with familial dysautonomia (FD) have abnormal ventilatory responses to hypoxia and hypercapnia, and in FD children, CSA is common. Sudden death in FD may be related to their abnormal ventilatory control.[150]

CSA has also been described in neuromuscular disorders such as Duchenne muscular dystrophy[151] and myotonic dystrophy.[152] Whether or not the CSA and abnormal ventilatory responses are due to muscular inability to mount thoracoabdominal movement or centrally mediated ventilatory dysregulation, nevertheless respiratory supportive treatment should take these findings into account.

Summary

CSA and hypoventilation in children can result from various structural and functional disorders that affect the brainstem or ventilatory control. Early recognition through PSG and neuroimaging is essential, as targeted treatment (eg, surgical, medical, or supportive ventilation) can greatly improve patient outcomes. Ongoing follow-up is crucial given the potential for persistent or progressive respiratory control abnormalities.

CLINICS CARE POINTS

- Gold Standard Diagnosis: A full-night in-laboratory PSG is the gold standard for diagnosing CSA, as the condition cannot be reliably diagnosed based on clinical history alone.
- Diagnostic Thresholds: Pathological CSA should be suspected when the CAI is > 5 events per hour. A higher CAI (>10 events per hour) is more likely to be associated with structural abnormalities on an MRI, such as Chiari malformations or brainstem tumors.
- Potential Underdiagnosis: Relying solely on the CAI may lead to underdiagnosis if central hypopneas are not also included in the diagnostic criteria.
- ROHHAD Misclassification: Since hypoventilation may not be present at the onset of rapid weight gain, ROHHAD can easily be misclassified as simple obesity, potentially delaying PSG surveillance.
- Emerging ROHHAD Biomarkers: The presence of ZSCAN1 autoantibodies has been identified as a potential candidate biomarker for ROHHAD, particularly in those with neuroblastic tumors.
- PWS Management: Low-flow oxygen is the primary treatment for CSA in infants with PWS. Most of these patients can be weaned off oxygen by two years of age as their breathing control matures.
- CCHS Genotype/Phenotype: In CCHS, longer polyalanine repeat mutations (PARMs) of the PHOX2b gene are associated with more severe hypoventilation requiring more daytime ventilatory support.
- The Use of Oxygen in CCHS: Using supplemental oxygen alone to treat CCHS is insufficient to treat the underlying hypoventilation and can worsen the condition by further depressing the respiratory drive.

DECLARATION OF AI AND AI-ASSISTED TECHNOLOGIES IN THE WRITING PROCESS

During the preparation of this work, the authors used Grammarly in order to proofread and suggest corrections. After using this tool/service, the authors reviewed and edited the content as needed and take full responsibility for the content of the publication.

DISCLOSURE

The authors have nothing to disclose.

REFERENCES

1. American Academy of Sleep Medicine. Central sleep apnea syndromes. In: International classification of sleep disorders. 3rd edition. American Academy of Sleep Medicine; 2014. p. 69–107.
2. Erickson G, Dobson NR, Hunt CE. Immature control of breathing and apnea of prematurity: the known and unknown. J Perinatol 2021;41(9):2111–23.
3. Troester MM, Quan SF, Berry RB, et al. The AASM manual for the scoring of sleep and associated events: rules, terminology and technical specifications. Version 3. American Academy of Sleep Medicine; 2023.
4. Kritzinger FE, Al-Saleh S, Narang I. Descriptive analysis of central sleep apnea in childhood at a single center. Pediatr Pulmonol 2011;46(10):1023–30.
5. McLaren AT, Bin-Hasan S, Narang I. Diagnosis, management and pathophysiology of central sleep apnea in children. Paediatr Respir Rev 2019;30:49–57.
6. Restrepo-Gualteros SM, Villamil-Osorio M, Rodriguez-Martinez CE. Prediction of normal values for central apnea-hypopnea index at different ages and altitudes above sea level in healthy children. Sleep Med 2021;78:182–8.
7. Wang G, Xu Z, Tai J, et al. Normative values of polysomnographic parameters in Chinese children and adolescents: a cross-sectional study. Sleep Med 2016;27-28:49–53.
8. Vézina K, Mariasine J, Young R, et al. Cardiorespiratory monitoring data during sleep in healthy Canadian infants. Annals ATS 2020;17(10):1238–46.
9. Montgomery-Downs HE, O'Brien LM, Gulliver TE, et al. Polysomnographic characteristics in normal preschool and early school-aged children. Pediatrics 2006;117(3):741–53.

10. Stowe RC, Miranda-Schaeubinger M, Andronikou S, et al. Polysomnographic predictors of abnormal brainstem imaging in children. J Clin Sleep Med 2021;17(7):1411–21.
11. Duenas-Meza E, Bazurto-Zapata MA, Gozal D, et al. Overnight polysomnographic characteristics and oxygen saturation of healthy infants, 1 to 18 months of age, born and residing at high altitude (2,640 meters). Chest 2015;148(1):120–7.
12. Tanphaichitr A, Tanphaichitr P, Apiwattanasawee P, et al. Prevalence and risk factors for central sleep apnea in infants with laryngomalacia. Otolaryngol Head Neck Surg 2014;150(4):677–83.
13. Cataldi M, Arnaldi D, Tucci V, et al. Sleep disorders in Prader-Willi syndrome, evidence from animal models and humans. Sleep Med Rev 2021;57: 101432. https://doi.org/10.1016/j.smrv.2021.101432.
14. Voutsas G, St-Laurent A, Hutchinson C, et al. The efficacy of neurosurgical intervention on sleep-disordered breathing in pediatric patients with Chiari malformation type I. J Neurosurg Pediatr 2021;27(6):611–9.
15. Felix O, Amaddeo A, Olmo Arroyo J, et al. Central sleep apnea in children: experience at a single center. Sleep Med 2016;25:24–8.
16. Amin R, Sharma N, Al-Mokali K, et al. Sleep-disordered breathing in children with chronic kidney disease. Pediatr Nephrol 2015;30(12):2135–43.
17. Albert GW. Chiari malformation in children. Pediatr Clin North Am 2021;68(4):783–92.
18. Combs D, Skrepnek G, Seckeler MD, et al. Sleep-disordered breathing is associated with increased mortality in hospitalized infants with congenital heart disease. J Clin Sleep Med 2018;14(09):1551–8.
19. Jain SV, Simakajornboon N, Arthur TM. Central sleep apnea: does stabilizing sleep improve it? J Child Neurol 2014;29(1):96–8.
20. Seppä-Moilanen M, Andersson S, Kirjavainen T. Caffeine is a respiratory stimulant without effect on sleep in the short-term in late-preterm infants. Pediatr Res 2022;92(3):776–82.
21. Xiao L, Sunkonkit K, Chiang J, et al. Unexplained significant central sleep apnea in infants: clinical presentation and outcomes. Sleep Breath 2023; 27(1):255–64.
22. Hayashi A, Suresh S, Kevat A, et al. Central sleep apnea in otherwise healthy term infants. J Clin Sleep Med 2022;18(12):2813–7.
23. Goldberg A. Clinical indications for noninvasive positive pressure ventilation in chronic respiratory failure due to restrictive lung disease, COPD, and nocturnal hypoventilation – a consensus conference report. Chest 1999;116(2):521–34.
24. Ferreira R, Lemos A, Oliveira L, et al. Sleep related hypoventilation: should the paediatric definition be revised? Eur Respir J 2020;56(suppl 64). https://doi.org/10.1183/13993003.congress-2020.1180.
25. Ross KR, Rosen CL. Sleep and respiratory physiology in children. Clin Chest Med 2014;35(3): 457–67.
26. Dudoignon B, Bokov P, Benterki F, et al. Reliability of composite autonomic symptom score (COMPASS)-31 in congenital central hypoventilation syndrome. Pediatr Pulmonol 2025;60(4):e71072. https://doi.org/10.1002/ppul.71072.
27. Weese-Mayer DE, Rand CM, Khaytin I, et al. Congenital central hypoventilation syndrome. In: Adam MP, Feldman J, Mirzaa GM, et al, editors. GeneReviews®. University of Washington, Seattle; 2021. Available at: http://www.ncbi.nlm.nih.gov/books/NBK1427/. Accessed October 8, 2025.
28. Trang H, Samuels M, Ceccherini I, et al. Guidelines for diagnosis and management of congenital central hypoventilation syndrome. Orphanet J Rare Dis 2020;15(1):252.
29. Jennings LJ, Yu M, Rand CM, et al. Variable human phenotype associated with novel deletions of the PHOX2B gene. Pediatr Pulmonol 2012; 47(2):153–61.
30. Amiel J, Laudier B, Attié-Bitach T, et al. Polyalanine expansion and frameshift mutations of the paired-like homeobox gene PHOX2B in congenital central hypoventilation syndrome. Nat Genet 2003;33(4): 459–61.
31. Weese-Mayer DE, Berry-Kravis EM, Zhou L, et al. Idiopathic congenital central hypoventilation syndrome: analysis of genes pertinent to early autonomic nervous system embryologic development and identification of mutations in PHOX2b. Am J Med Genet 2003;123A(3):267–78.
32. Sasaki A, Kanai M, Kijima K, et al. Molecular analysis of congenital central hypoventilation syndrome. Hum Genet 2003;114(1):22–6.
33. Sritippayawan S, Hamutcu R, Kun SS, et al. Mother–daughter transmission of congenital central hypoventilation syndrome. Am J Respir Crit Care Med 2002;166(3):367–9.
34. Silvestri JM, Chen ML, Weese-Mayer DE, et al. Idiopathic congenital central hypoventilation syndrome: the next generation. Am J Med Genet 2002;112(1): 46–50.
35. Huang J, Colrain IM, Panitch HB, et al. Effect of sleep stage on breathing in children with central hypoventilation. J Appl Physiol 2008;105(1): 44–53.
36. Zelko FA, Welbel RZ, Rand CM, et al. Neurocognition as a biomarker in the rare autonomic disorders of CCHS and ROHHAD. Clin Auton Res 2023; 33(3):217–30.
37. Hino A, Terada J, Kasai H, et al. Adult cases of late-onset congenital central hypoventilation syndrome and paired-like homeobox 2B-mutation carriers: an additional case report and pooled analysis. J Clin Sleep Med 2020;16(11):1891–900.

38. Dudoignon B, Peters J, Paglietti MG, et al. European central hypoventilation syndrome consortium description of congenital central hypoventilation syndrome neonatal onset. Eur J Pediatr 2025; 184(2):161.
39. Meguro T, Yoshida Y, Hayashi M, et al. Inheritance of polyalanine expansion mutation of PHOX2B in congenital central hypoventilation syndrome. J Hum Genet 2012;57(5):335–7.
40. Laifman E, Keens TG, Bar-Cohen Y, et al. Life-threatening cardiac arrhythmias in congenital central hypoventilation syndrome. Eur J Pediatr 2020; 179(5):821–5.
41. Balakrishnan K, Perez IA, Keens TG, et al. Hirschsprung disease and other gastrointestinal motility disorders in patients with CCHS. Eur J Pediatr 2021;180(2):469–73.
42. Trang H, Bourgeois P, Cheliout-Heraut F. Neurocognition in congenital central hypoventilation syndrome: influence of genotype and ventilation method. Orphanet J Rare Dis 2020;15(1):322.
43. Weese-Mayer DE, Berry-Kravis EM, Ceccherini I, et al. An official ATS clinical policy statement: congenital central hypoventilation syndrome. Am J Respir Crit Care Med 2010;181(6):626–44.
44. Byers HM, Chen M, Gelfand AS, et al. Expanding the phenotype of congenital central hypoventilation syndrome impacts management decisions. Am J Med Genet 2018;176(6):1398–404.
45. Kasi AS, Jurgensen TJ, Yen S, et al. Three-generation family with congenital central hypoventilation syndrome and novel PHOX2B gene non-polyalanine repeat mutation. J Clin Sleep Med 2017;13(07): 925–7.
46. Katwa U, D'Gama AM, Qualls AE, et al. Atypical presentations associated with non-polyalanine repeat PHOX2B mutations. Am J Med Genet 2018;176(7): 1627–31.
47. Zhou A, Rand CM, Hockney SM, et al. Paired-like homeobox gene (*PHOX2B*) nonpolyalanine repeat expansion mutations (NPARMs): genotype–phenotype correlation in congenital central hypoventilation syndrome (CCHS). Genet Med 2021; 23(9):1656–63.
48. Zelko FA, Stewart TM, Brogadir CD, et al. Weese-Mayer DE. Congenital central hypoventilation syndrome: broader cognitive deficits revealed by parent controls. Pediatr Pulmonol 2018;53(4): 492–7.
49. Gozal D, Keens TG. Passive nighttime hypocapnic hyperventilation improves daytime eucapnia in mechanically ventilated children. Am J Respir Crit Care Med 1998;157(3):A779.
50. Barlow PB, Bartlett D, Hauri P, et al. Idiopathic hypoventilation syndrome: importance of preventing nocturnal hypoxemia and hypercapnia. Am Rev Respir Dis 1980;121(1):141–5.
51. Straus C, Trang H, Becquemin MH, et al. Chemosensitivity recovery in Ondine's curse syndrome under treatment with desogestrel. Respir Physiol Neurobiol 2010;171(2):171–4.
52. Schirwani S, Pysden K, Chetcuti P, et al. Carbamazepine improves apneic episodes in Congenital Central Hypoventilation Syndrome (CCHS) with a novel PHOX2B exon 1 missense mutation. J Clin Sleep Med 2017;13(11):1359–62.
53. Mathur S, Laifman E, Keens TG, et al. Children with congenital central hypoventilation syndrome do not wake up to ventilator alarms. Sleep Breath 2022; 26(3):1277–80.
54. Basu SM, Chung FF, AbdelHakim SF, et al. Anesthetic considerations for patients with congenital central hypoventilation syndrome: a systematic review of the literature. Anesth Analg 2017; 124(1):169.
55. Khayat A, Medin D, Syed F, et al. Intelligent volume-assured pressured support (iVAPS) for the treatment of congenital central hypoventilation syndrome. Sleep Breath 2017;21(2):513–9.
56. Maloney MA, Kun SS, Keens TG, et al. Congenital central hypoventilation syndrome: diagnosis and management. Exp Rev Respir Med 2018;12(4): 283–92.
57. Roberts SD, Kapadia H, Greenlee G, et al. Midfacial and dental changes associated with nasal positive airway pressure in children with obstructive sleep apnea and craniofacial conditions. J Clin Sleep Med 2016;12(04):469–75.
58. Tibballs J, Henning RD. Noninvasive ventilatory strategies in the management of a newborn infant and three children with congenital central hypoventilation syndrome. Pediatr Pulmonol 2003;36(6): 544–8.
59. Xu Z, Wu Y, Li B, et al. Noninvasive ventilation in a young infant with congenital central hypoventilation and 7-year follow-up. Pediatr Investig 2019;03(04): 261–4.
60. Kasi AS, Anand N, Harford KL, et al. Tracheostomy decannulation to noninvasive positive pressure ventilation in congenital central hypoventilation syndrome. Sleep Breath 2022;26(1):133–9.
61. Paglietti MG, Porcaro F, Sovtic A, et al. Decannulation in children affected by congenital central hypoventilation syndrome: a proposal of an algorithm from two European centers. Pediatr Pulmonol 2019;54(11):1663–9.
62. Hartmann H, Samuels MP, Noyes JP, et al. Negative extrathoracic pressure ventilation in infants and young children with central hypoventilation syndrome. Pediatr Pulmonol 1997;23(2):155–7.
63. Marcus CL, Jansen MT, Poulsen MK, et al. Medical and psychosocial outcome of children with congenital central hypoventilation syndrome. J Pediatr 1991;119(6):888–95.

64. Chen ML, Tablizo MA, Kun S, et al. Diaphragm pacers as a treatment for congenital central hypoventilation syndrome. Expert Rev Med Dev 2005; 2(5):577–85.
65. Nicholson KJ, Nosanov LB, Bowen KA, et al. Thoracoscopic placement of phrenic nerve pacers for diaphragm pacing in congenital central hypoventilation syndrome. J Pediatr Surg 2015;50(1):78–81.
66. Diaphragm Pacemakers - The Avery Diaphragm Pacing System. Avery biomedical. Available at: https://averybiomedical.com/diaphragm-pacing-system/. Accessed October 8, 2025.
67. Maloney MA, Keens TG, Vanderlaan MB, et al. Pregnancy in congenital central hypoventilation syndrome. Am J Obstet Gynecol MFM 2020;2(4): 100237. https://doi.org/10.1016/j.ajogmf.2020.100237.
68. Duty BD, Wozniak SE, Selden NR. Vagal nerve stimulator placement for medically refractory seizures in a child treated with phrenic nerve pacing for congenital central hypoventilation syndrome: case report. J Neurosurg Pediatr 2011;7(4):413–5.
69. Kwon A, Lodge M, McComb JG, et al. An unusual cause of diaphragm pacer failure in congenital central hypoventilation syndrome. J Clin Sleep Med 2022;18(3):949–52.
70. Valika T, Chin AC, Thompson DM, et al. Airway obstruction during sleep due to diaphragm pacing precludes decannulation in young children with CCHS. Respiration 2019;98(3):263–7.
71. Diep B, Wang A, Kun S, et al. Diaphragm pacing without tracheostomy in congenital central hypoventilation syndrome patients. Respiration 2015; 89(6):534–8.
72. Wang A, Kun S, Diep B, et al. Obstructive sleep apnea in patients with congenital central hypoventilation syndrome ventilated by diaphragm pacing without tracheostomy. J Clin Sleep Med 2018;14-(02):261–4.
73. Tsolakis N, Sindelar R, Markström A, et al. Strategy of changing from tracheostomy and non-invasive mechanical ventilation to diaphragm pacing in children with congenital central hypoventilation syndrome. Acta Paediatr 2022;111(6):1245–7.
74. Fishman LS, Samson JH, Sperling DR. Primary alveolar hypoventilation syndrome (ondine's curse): association with manifestations of hypothalmic disease. Am J Dis Child 1965;110(2):155–61.
75. Ize-Ludlow D, Gray JA, Sperling MA, et al. Rapid-onset obesity with hypothalamic dysfunction, hypoventilation, and autonomic dysregulation presenting in childhood. Pediatrics 2007;120(1):e179–88.
76. Lee JM, Shin J, Kim S, et al. Rapid-onset obesity with hypoventilation, hypothalamic, autonomic dysregulation, and neuroendocrine tumors (ROHHAD-NET) syndrome: a systematic review. Biomed Res Int 2018;2018(1):1250721. https://doi.org/10.1155/2018/1250721.
77. Harvengt J, Gernay C, Mastouri M, et al. ROHHAD(NET) syndrome: systematic review of the clinical timeline and recommendations for diagnosis and prognosis. J Clin Endocrinol Metab 2020; 105(7):2119–31.
78. Khaytin I, Stewart TM, Zelko FA, et al. Evolution of physiologic and autonomic phenotype in rapid-onset obesity with hypothalamic dysfunction, hypoventilation, and autonomic dysregulation over a decade from age at diagnosis. J Clin Sleep Med 2022;18(3):937–44.
79. Lazea C, Sur L, Florea M. ROHHAD (Rapid-onset obesity with hypoventilation, hypothalamic dysfunction, autonomic dysregulation) syndrome—what every pediatrician should know about the etiopathogenesis, diagnosis and treatment: a review. Int J Gen Med 2021;14:319–26.
80. Khaytin I, Victor AK, Barclay SF, et al. Rapid-onset obesity with hypothalamic dysfunction, hypoventilation, and autonomic dysregulation (ROHHAD): a collaborative review of the current understanding. Clin Auton Res 2023;33(3):251–68.
81. Rand CM, Patwari PP, Rodikova EA, et al. Rapid-onset obesity with hypothalamic dysfunction, hypoventilation, and autonomic dysregulation: analysis of hypothalamic and autonomic candidate genes. Pediatr Res 2011;70(4):375–8.
82. Patwari PP, Wolfe LF. Rapid-onset obesity with hypothalamic dysfunction, hypoventilation, and autonomic dysregulation: review and update. Curr Opin Pediatr 2014;26(4):487.
83. Reppucci D, Hamilton J, Yeh EA, et al. ROHHAD syndrome and evolution of sleep disordered breathing. Orphanet J Rare Dis 2016;11(1):106.
84. Bougnères P, Pantalone L, Linglart A, et al. Endocrine manifestations of the rapid-onset obesity with hypoventilation, hypothalamic, autonomic dysregulation, and neural tumor syndrome in childhood. J Clin Endocrinol Metab 2008;93(10): 3971–80.
85. Özcan G, Özsu E, Şiklar Z, et al. A rare cause of sleep-disordered breathing: ROHHAD syndrome. Front Pediatr 2020;8. https://doi.org/10.3389/fped.2020.573227.
86. Hawton K, Hilliard T, Langton-Hewer SC, et al. Rapid-onset obesity, hypothalamic dysfunction, hypoventilation, and autonomic dysregulation syndrome – neuro-endocrine tumours (ROHHAD-NET): case series and learning points. J Pediatr Endocrinol Metab 2023;36(4):418–23.
87. Dhondt K, Verloo P, Verhelst H, et al. Hypocretin-1 deficiency in a girl with ROHHAD syndrome. Pediatrics 2013;132(3):e788–92.
88. Selvadurai S, Benzon D, Voutsas G, et al. Sleep-disordered breathing, respiratory patterns during wakefulness and functional capacity in pediatric patients with rapid-onset obesity with hypothalamic dysfunction,

hypoventilation and autonomic dysregulation syndrome. Pediatr Pulmonol 2021;56(2):479–85.
89. Filippidou M, Petropoulou T, Botsa E, et al. ROHHAD syndrome – a still unrecognized cause of childhood obesity: report of three cases. J Pediatr Endocrinol Metab 2020;33(10):1341–8.
90. Carroll MS, Patwari PP, Kenny AS, et al. Rapid-onset obesity with hypothalamic dysfunction, hypoventilation, and autonomic dysregulation (ROHHAD): response to ventilatory challenges. Pediatr Pulmonol 2015;50(12):1336–45.
91. Guyenet PG. Regulation of breathing and autonomic outflows by chemoreceptors. Compr Physiol 2014;4(4):1511–62.
92. Forster HV, Haouzi P, Dempsey JA. Control of breathing during exercise. Compr Physiol 2012;2(1):743–77.
93. Burton DA, Stokes K, Hall GM. Physiological effects of exercise. Cont Educ Anaesth Crit Care Pain 2004;4(6):185–8.
94. Milla CE, Zirbes J. Pulmonary complications of endocrine and metabolic disorders. Paediatr Respir Rev 2012;13(1):23–8.
95. Powers SK, Beadle RE. Control of ventilation during submaximal exercise: a brief review. J Sports Sci 1985;3(1):51–65.
96. Patwari PP, Rand CM, Berry-Kravis EM, et al. Monozygotic twins discordant for ROHHAD phenotype. Pediatrics 2011;128(3):e711–5.
97. Barclay SF, Rand CM, Gray PA, et al. Absence of mutations in *HCRT, HCRTR1* and *HCRTR2* in patients with ROHHAD. Respir Physiol Neurobiol 2016;221:59–63.
98. Barclay SF, Rand CM, Borch LA, et al. Rapid-onset obesity with hypothalamic dysfunction, hypoventilation, and autonomic dysregulation (ROHHAD): exome sequencing of trios, monozygotic twins and tumours. Orphanet J Rare Dis 2015;10(1):103.
99. Giacomozzi C, Guaraldi F, Cambiaso P, et al. Anti-hypothalamus and anti-pituitary auto-antibodies in ROHHAD syndrome: additional evidence supporting an autoimmune etiopathogenesis. Horm Res Paediatr 2019;92(2):124–32.
100. Jacobson LA, Rane S, McReynolds LJ, et al. Improved behavior and neuropsychological function in children with ROHHAD after high-dose cyclophosphamide. Pediatrics 2016;138(1):e20151080. https://doi.org/10.1542/peds.2015-1080.
101. Mandel-Brehm C, Benson LA, Tran B, et al. ZSCAN1 autoantibodies are associated with pediatric paraneoplastic ROHHAD. Ann Neurol 2022;92(2):279–91.
102. Stowe RC, Afolabi-Brown O. Pulmonary hypertension and chronic hypoventilation in ROHHAD syndrome treated with average-volume assured pressure support. Pediatr Investig 2019;03(04):253–6.
103. Katz ES, McGrath S, Marcus CL. Late-onset central hypoventilation with hypothalamic dysfunction: a distinct clinical syndrome. Pediatr Pulmonol 2000;29(1):62–8.
104. Jalal Eldin AW, Tombayoglu D, Butz L, et al. Natural history of ROHHAD syndrome: development of severe insulin resistance and fatty liver disease over time. Clin Diabetes Endocrinol 2019;5(1):9.
105. Cassidy SB, Dykens E, Williams CA. Prader-willi and angelman syndromes: sister imprinted disorders. Am J Med Genet 2000;97(2):136–46.
106. Butler MG, Hartin SN, Hossain WA, et al. Molecular genetic classification in Prader-Willi syndrome: a multisite cohort study. J Med Genet 2019;56(3):149–53.
107. Driscoll DJ, Miller JL, Cassidy SB. Prader-willi syndrome. In: Adam MP, Feldman J, Mirzaa GM, et al, editors. GeneReviews®. University of Washington, Seattle; 1993. Available at: http://www.ncbi.nlm.nih.gov/books/NBK1330/. Accessed October 9, 2025.
108. Hartin SN, Hossain WA, Francis D, et al. Analysis of the Prader–Willi syndrome imprinting center using droplet digital PCR and next-generation whole-exome sequencing. Mol Genet Genom Med 2019;7(4):e00575. https://doi.org/10.1002/mgg3.575.
109. Deal CL, Tony M, Höybye C, et al. The 2011 growth hormone in Prader-Willi syndrome clinical care guidelines workshop participants. Growth hormone research society workshop summary: Consensus guidelines for recombinant human growth hormone therapy in Prader-Willi syndrome. J Clin Endocrinol Metab 2013;98(6):E1072–87.
110. Grugni G, Marzullo P. Diagnosis and treatment of GH deficiency in Prader–Willi syndrome. Best Pract Res Clin Endocrinol Metabol 2016;30(6):785–94.
111. Bridges N. What is the value of growth hormone therapy in prader willi syndrome? Arch Dis Child 2014;99(2):166–70.
112. Arens R, Gozal D, Burrell BC, et al. Arousal and cardiorespiratory responses to hypoxia in Prader-Willi syndrome. Am J Respir Crit Care Med 1996;153(1):283–7.
113. Cohen M, Hamilton J, Narang I. Clinically important age-related differences in sleep related disordered breathing in infants and children with Prader-Willi syndrome. PLoS One 2014;9(6):e101012. https://doi.org/10.1371/journal.pone.0101012.
114. Sedky K, Bennett DS, Pumariega A. Prader Willi syndrome and obstructive sleep apnea: co-Occurrence in the pediatric population. J Clin Sleep Med 2014;10(04):403–9.
115. Tan YT, Azanan MS, Hng SY, et al. Long-term effect of growth hormone on sleep-disordered breathing in Malaysian children with Prader-Willi syndrome: a retrospective study. J Clin Sleep Med 2024;20(8):1291–9.
116. Oboleviciene G, Vaideliene L, Miseviciene V. Exploring sleep-related breathing disorders in

pediatric obesity and Prader-Willi syndrome. Respir Med 2024;234:107855. https://doi.org/10.1016/j.rmed.2024.107855.
117. Schaefer J, Davey MJ, Nixon GM. Sleep-disordered breathing in school-aged children with Prader-Willi syndrome. J Clin Sleep Med 2022; 18(4):1055–61.
118. Omokawa M, Ayabe T, Nagai T, et al. Decline of CSF orexin (hypocretin) levels in Prader–Willi syndrome. Am J Med Genet 2016;170(5):1181–6.
119. de Lind van Wijngaarden RFA, Joosten KFM, van den Berg S, et al. The relationship between central adrenal insufficiency and sleep-related breathing disorders in children with Prader-Willi syndrome. J Clin Endocrinol Metab 2009;94(7):2387–93.
120. Gozal D, Arens R, Omlin KJ, et al. Absent peripheral chemosensitivity in Prader-Willi syndrome. J Appl Physiol 1994;77(5):2231–6.
121. Arens R, Gozal D, Omlin KJ, et al. Hypoxic and hypercapnic ventilatory responses in Prader-Willi syndrome. J Appl Physiol 1994;77(5):2224–30.
122. Urquhart DS, Gulliver T, Williams G, et al. Central sleep-disordered breathing and the effects of oxygen therapy in infants with Prader-Willi syndrome. Arch Dis Child 2013;98(8):592–5.
123. Khayat A, Narang I, Bin-Hasan S, et al. Longitudinal evaluation of sleep disordered breathing in infants with Prader-Willi syndrome. Arch Dis Child 2017;102(7):634–8.
124. Smith IE, King MA, Siklos PW, et al. Treatment of ventilatory failure in the Prader-Willi syndrome. Eur Respir J 1998;11(5):1150–2.
125. Dauvilliers Y, Arnulf I, Szakacs Z, et al. HARMONY III study group. Long-term use of pitolisant to treat patients with narcolepsy: harmony III study. Sleep 2019;42(11):zsz174.
126. DeCock VC, Diene G, Molinas C, et al. Efficacy of modafinil on excessive daytime sleepiness in Prader–Willi syndrome. Am J Med Genet 2011; 155(7):1552–7.
127. Pennington S, Stutzman D, Sannar E. Pitolisant in an adolescent with Prader-Willi syndrome. J Pediatr Pharmacol Therapeut 2021;26(4):405–10.
128. Rosen G, Brand SR. Sleep in children with cancer: case review of 70 children evaluated in a comprehensive pediatric sleep center. Support Care Cancer 2011;19(7):985–94.
129. Helligsoe ASL, Weile KS, Kenborg L, et al. Systematic review: sleep disorders based on objective data in children and adolescents treated for a brain tumor. Front Neurosci 2022;16:808398. https://doi.org/10.3389/fnins.2022.808398.
130. Mandrell BN, Wise M, Schoumacher RA, et al. Excessive daytime sleepiness and sleep-disordered breathing disturbances in survivors of childhood central nervous system tumors. Pediatr Blood Cancer 2012;58(5):746–51.
131. Fujimoto K, Kasai H, Kunii R, et al. Obstructive sleep apnea in a severely Obese child with combined central sleep apnea and sleep-related hypoventilation disorder caused by a medullary tumor. J Clin Sleep Med 2018;14(06):1071–4.
132. Cordani R, Veneruso M, Napoli F, et al. Sleep disturbances in pediatric craniopharyngioma: a systematic review. Front Neurol 2022;13:876011. https://doi.org/10.3389/fneur.2022.876011.
133. Huang SW, Lee PL, Fan PC, et al. Diffuse midline glioma presenting with central sleep apnea and pulmonary hypertension in a 4-year-old patient: a case report. J Clin Sleep Med 2021;17(2):325–8.
134. Ju Wang JD, Doherty D, Ramirez JM, et al. Central sleep apnea in patients with pontine tegmental cap dysplasia treated with supplemental oxygen: a case report. J Clin Sleep Med 2023;19(4):843–9.
135. Ju-Wang JD, Dempsey JC, Zhang C, et al. Sleep and breathing in children with Joubert syndrome and a review of other rare congenital hindbrain malformations. Ther Adv Respir Dis 2025;19: 17534666241308405. https://doi.org/10.1177/17534666241308405.
136. Fauroux B, AlSayed M, Ben-Omran T, et al. Management of sleep-disordered breathing in achondroplasia: guiding principles of the european achondroplasia forum. Orphanet J Rare Dis 2025; 20(1):233.
137. Costa F, Ait Benali S, Dantas F, et al. Chiari malformation: diagnosis, classifications, natural history, and conservative management. World Federation of neurosurgical societies spine committee recommendations. Spine 2025;50(11):767–78.
138. Leu RM. Sleep-related breathing disorders and the chiari 1 malformation. Chest 2015;148(5):1346–52.
139. Kirjavainen T, Miraftabi P, Martelius L, et al. Type one Chiari malformation as a cause of central sleep apnea and hypoventilation in children. Sleep Med 2024;116:32–40.
140. Strang A, Katwa U. Persistent central apnea and long-term outcome after posterior fossa decompressive surgery for Arnold Chiari type 1 malformation in a pediatric patient. J Clin Sleep Med 2019; 15(04):667–71.
141. Waters KA, Forbes P, Morielli A, et al. Sleep-disordered breathing in children with myelomeningocele. J Pediatr 1998;132(4):672–81.
142. Patel DM, Rocque BG, Hopson B, et al. Sleep-disordered breathing in patients with myelomeningocele. J Neurosurg Pediatr 2015;16(1):30–5.
143. Shellhaas RA, Kenia PV, Hassan F, et al. Sleep-disordered breathing among newborns with myelomeningocele. J Pediatr 2018;194:244–7.e1.
144. Jernigan SC, Berry JG, Graham DA, et al. Risk factors of sudden death in young adult patients with myelomeningocele. J Neurosurg Pediatr 2012; 9(2):149–55.

145. Antics D, Kelemen JN, Muzslay E, et al. Nocturnal hypoventilation in children with obesity. Sleep Med 2025;134:106748. https://doi.org/10.1016/j.sleep.2025.106748.
146. Alves CAPF, Teixeira SR, Martin-Saavedra JS, et al. Pediatric leigh syndrome: neuroimaging features and genetic correlations. Ann Neurol 2020;88(2):218–32.
147. Chang X, Wu Y, Zhou J, et al. A meta-analysis and systematic review of Leigh syndrome: clinical manifestations, respiratory chain enzyme complex deficiency, and gene mutations. Medicine (Baltim) 2020;99(5):e18634. https://doi.org/10.1097/MD.0000000000018634.
148. Ju Wang JD, Chen M, Zhang C, et al. Sleep and breathing disturbances in children with Leigh syndrome: a comparative study. Pediatr Neurol 2022;136:56–63.
149. Sofou K, De Coo IFM, Isohanni P, et al. A multicenter study on Leigh syndrome: disease course and predictors of survival. Orphanet J Rare Dis 2014;9:52.
150. Palma JA, Gileles-Hillel A, Norcliffe-Kaufmann L, et al. Chemoreflex failure and sleep-disordered breathing in familial dysautonomia: implications for sudden death during sleep. Auton Neurosci 2019;218:10–5.
151. Sawnani H, Thampratankul L, Szczesniak RD, et al. Sleep disordered breathing in young boys with Duchenne muscular dystrophy. J Pediatr 2015;166(3):640–5.e1.
152. Hawkins AM, Hawkins CL, Abdul Razak K, et al. Respiratory dysfunction in myotonic dystrophy type 1: a systematic review. Neuromuscul Disord 2019;29(3):198–212.

9780443470448